W

Saying About This Book

If you want to get moving in your spiritual walk, try reading Lisa's transformational approach to prayer. Watch her life change as she combines prayer and honesty in a way that brings her healing and blesses those around her. Reading her stories brings prayer to life – it's a way of combining being real with being faithful which is life-transforming. If you feel that your stuff is blocking your relationship with God, or you want some help battling your emotions, or you just want to try a way of praying that is more integrated read Real Talk with God.

—Mike Jones, St Mary's Centre for Peace and Reconciliation and Vicar of Luton, U.K.

Pinkham's book can be read like a devotional with each portion taking the reader into their God-given imagination in dealing with common life hardships and relatable joy-filled moments. Like a play with narrative and dialogue, there are scenes and exchanges that will be with me for a long time (like the three-legged race), informing my relationship with God and others for good. Often light and humorous, frequently deep and impacting, this book is a keeper as a reminder that God is desirous of conversation in every thought, feeling and situation. Without pretense or preachiness, words from the Bible are woven throughout and brought to light in her conversations. Jump-start your heart-to-heart exchanges with God with this accessible model.

—Christine Bender, Inveterate Pursuer of God,
Western Washington State

The author faces and processes many complex emotions that many people would run from by engaging with God, getting God's perspective and quieting her soul. This is a powerful book for anyone who struggles with negative emotions and doesn't know what to do.

—Betsy Stalcup, Founder and Executive
Director of Healing Center International
author of Facing Life's Losses, Whispers in the
Storm and Immanuel: Enjoying God's Presence
(DVD) https://www.godhealstoday.org

Lisa is a masterful storyteller. That gift coupled with her tenacious pursuit of God's perspective and presence offers the world hope and peace in the midst of internal chaos, relational breakdown, and even trauma. A must read for anyone struggling to find light in the darkness.

—Toni M. Daniels, author of Back to
Joy, Training Consultant for Godly Play
Communitas and LK10

Our brains change when we see a model of who we want to become. Lisa Pinkham's REAL TALK WITH GOD offers you a beautiful display of a real human interaction with our Real God. The world needs more people like Lisa and this book is a gift to anyone seeking a life with God.

—John Loppnow, Marriage and Family Therapist, co-author of Joyful Journey, https://loppnowrelationshipcenter.com, www.PresenceAndPractice.com

Jesus speaks to us. Don't believe me? Read this book.

—Tony, businessman, Ireland

Do you sometimes feel like God is far away? Do you want to experience life-changing conversations with God in your daily life? If so, you should read Real Talk with God by Lisa Pinkham. By sharing her authentic conversations with God, the author introduces us to a more intimate, deep and personal way of talking with God. This amazing book will refresh your prayer life and lead you on a life-giving journey of self-discovery through communion with God.

—Myung Eun Park, Pastor of Readfield United Methodist Church, Maine

An excellent guide to a deep, conversational prayer life! Real Talk with God is based on the premises "that we can know and be known by a personal God who created us, walked in our shoes." It helps readers get out of their own heads and have honest conversations with God. Honest, real, and based on the author's personal experiences, Real Talk with God provides a roadmap for a deeper prayer life. The author does an excellent job of modeling conversational prayer, and I recommend this book to anyone wanting a more personal prayer life!

—Jed Jurchenko, Psychology Professor, Therapist, Coach and Author

A life-changing read! 'Real Talk with God' had me captivated from the beginning. At every step of the way I kept thinking of people I know who would be blessed by going on this journey -- a journey that speaks of hope and real intimacy with God.

—Jen Hamilton, disciple-maker, Thailand and Australia

In this book Real Talk, Lisa offers you the warmth of friendship and the comfort of a safe embrace as she invites you into another world. A world that opens you up to wholeness like you've not known before. A world where you and I can have an intimate two-way relationship with Christ! You will smile and may even cry as you experience a deep sense of gratitude and will enjoy the gentle and tender guidance that instructs you as you go down a path least traveled.

—Leona Njoku-Obi, Spiritual Formation Assistant, Marriage Coach, Concord, California

It has truly been a joy to peer into Lisa's journey with God and glean from her insights on how we too can have a "Real Talk With God"!

—Atara McGill, marketplace mentor, Virginia

This book is a collection of intimate and thoughtful conversations with God that Lisa has had over several years tracing her journey of seeking God in a wide variety of situations. She is honest about her struggles and weaknesses, yet tenacious in holding on to her belief that God has something good for her even in stressful, difficult times. It is not an autobiography in that the primary purpose of the book is not to tell us her story, but she uses her story to encourage us as readers to likewise engage in conversations with God, allowing us to see hers as models for us. Having read her conversations, I feel invited (by her? by God?) to follow her lead in seeking a more vital life with God.

—William Cutler, Intervarsity Christian Fellowship, New England

Lisa's writing launched me into worship and a very tender moment with God. I believe it will open up pathways for people to God. Those that honor Lisa's writings will get the impartation of her quality connection to God. I am excited for the readers and myself to go deeper in God. Soooo good.

—Mina Millen, Associate Marriage & Family Therapist and Professional Clinical Counselor, California

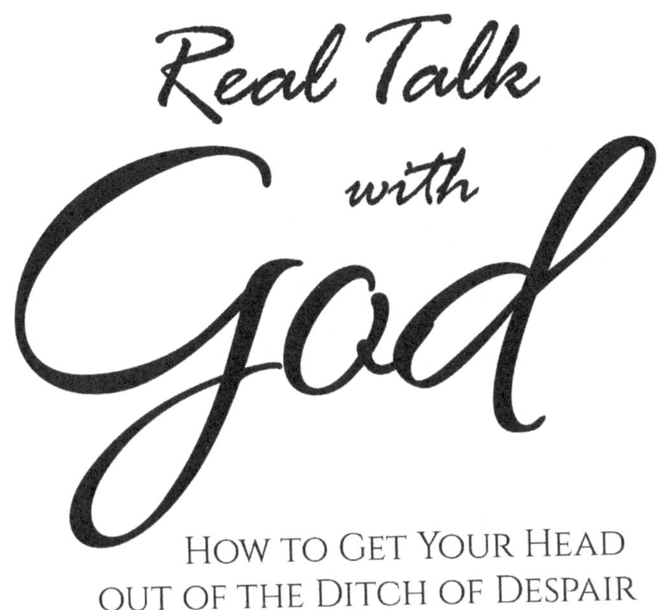

HOW TO GET YOUR HEAD OUT OF THE DITCH OF DESPAIR

LISA DODGE PINKHAM

Real Talk with God: How to Get Your Head out of the Ditch of Despair.

lisadodgepinkham@gmail.com

ISBN (paperback): 978-0-692-03610-5

Cover design and interior formatting: Matias Baldanza, for Chasing Kites Publishing.

Dedication

To Anita and all those who have served in the military...

Thank you for your service and sacrifice to our country and for still paying daily for our freedom.

I honor you.

Contents

Introduction

"I feel completely alone. My life seems utterly worthless. What purpose do I have in staying on this planet?" Did I actually just say this out loud? How did I ever get to this place? After thirty hours of emotional disorientation and at the end of a two-hour drive, I found myself completely consumed by these thoughts. My car may have still been on the road, but my head was stuck in a ditch. Shocked and bewildered at the intensity of my despair, I desperately scanned the long list of people who knew me, wondering who I could hang out with while I tried to get myself back on track.

How could there not be a single person in my contact list whom I could turn to without worrying that I would be too much for them or that they would be too much for me, doing more harm than good?

These thoughts totally drowned out any connection I had with God. It seemed as if the One who created me, who had been in my life for over thirty years had quietly slipped out without even saying goodbye. If I didn't have God, and I didn't have others, to whom could I turn? How could I go on with life?

I took a detour and headed for a church that was hosting a twelve-hour open house with local musicians playing worship music. I expected to unobtrusively slip into a corner, sing a little, and reconnect with myself and God. Instead, someone I knew approached me and said she had a prayer she wanted to say for me. Although she did wait for my consent to be prayed for, I felt worse after she finished than I did in my car. What could I possibly do next?

I called my parents and said between sobs, *"I am having a really rough day. I can't talk about it yet, but would you please just tell me some stories about your new cat? I know you are enjoying her, and she reminds me of the cat we had when I was in high school."* The only thing that made sense to me in that meltdown was that I needed to hear a joyful story that somehow connected my past to my present so that I could feel some hope for the future. I did feel better after hearing their stories, and I was able to think more clearly, implementing small action steps to rest and care for myself that day and in the days to come.

My intuition about what I needed eventually became my template for interacting with God. I learned how to get unstuck from negativity and practiced those skills with others. Most of all, I unlocked my heart and came clean with God about my thoughts, feelings, and needs. As a result, I discovered afresh how much He values me and wants me to live a vibrant and adventurous life.

Now I feel peaceful being with God, and I feel joyful knowing that He is with me. I have learned how to stay in a conversation and keep it real with Him, even, and especially, when I feel confused, sad, ashamed, angry, or afraid. And similar to my parents' cat stories, I have heard Him tell me stories that connected my past with my present, giving me hope for the future.

If you could see a before and after picture of my heart, it would look like a scrawny ragamuffin turned award-winning bodybuilder. My inner drive to overcome anxiety and despondency has culminated in a greater vitality and purpose than I thought possible, especially now that I am in my fifties. I relentlessly integrated my education, training, and experiences for my own transformation. Now I enthusiastically coach those who are motivated to get out of their own ditches, access their true selves, and have maximum impact with their lives.

I find myself and those I hang out with laughing, appreciating life, and sharing it with God. We marvel at our curiosity and patience when attacked by challenges. The blank, dark spots of our personal timelines are filled in and illuminated with positive memories and awareness of God's faithful interactions. Partnerships with God and our best, true selves are yielding clear thinking and confident decision-making. As we share this way of relating to God with others, especially during painful and confusing circumstances, our energy and sense of purpose is continually renewed.

I have coaching clients and friends who come to me when they feel stressed, anxious, and overwhelmed with circumstances in their lives. Now, instead of venting, praying half-heartedly, or inflating our *"should do"* list, they ask if we can do our *"usual thing."* Together, we practice relaxing, talk briefly about how we are feeling, ask God to help us remember feeling joy and peace in our past and interact with Him about our present situations. With our perspectives reframed, we emerge with energy, clarity, and increased resilience. Clients who are managing anxiety depression, and PTSD have said:

"I am healthier than I ever thought I could be. I like God. I like myself."

"I am grateful for what I received from you. I have connected God with every decade of my life to today. I have found new goals to strive for with God in present day and daily use."

"I have tried everything for years, and this has worked better than anything else."

~~~

I hope that as you read this book, your own joy, peace, and sense of being known by God will be ignited. If we were neighbors, we might share these stories around a meal, on a walk, or while doing chores. A book will have to suffice for now. Please start here. Make time now. Stay with me in this moment before searching elsewhere. Embrace the idea that you have everything you need to talk and listen to God intimately and authentically right now. All you need is:

- a few minutes to relax your body (this helps quiet your mind).
- a mind that is open to gleaning new ideas from my conversations.
- a heart willing to fully engage and feel a little pain before it shifts into joy and peace.
- a journal to experiment with and jot down your reflections.
- curiosity about who God is and how He feels about you.

The conversations throughout this book are arranged by chapters, which reveal how I got back *on the road again*—from:

- paralyzed to deliberate
- confused to confident
- hidden to authentic
- ambivalent to alive
- prideful to teachable
- self-sufficient to vulnerable
- protective to adventurous
~~~

Do you want to travel through life with the qualities on the right side of these bullet points (deliberate, confident, authentic, etc.)? Join me, and witness how talking and listening to God changed how I deal with anxiety, depression, toxic shame, and negativity. It has restored and developed a deeper intimacy with Him and others. I want you to experience this in your life too.

I want you to:

- feel validated and valuable.
- know that you are admired and cherished by your Creator.
- know that your Creator wants you to live into your best, true self as much (and probably more) than you do.
- experience that God will always happily stay with you, no matter what.

~~~

As you listen in on my conversations with God and hear my stories, you will naturally absorb ideas about how to cultivate your own authentic conversations with God. My intent in writing this book is to model something that you can try for yourself, even if you don't have the time or money for additional resources. I demonstrate:

- *how to* pay attention to your emotions and your body.
- *how to* be real with God.
- *how to* keep an authentic conversation going when you feel like giving up.
- *how to* notice where God is, what He wants you to know, and how He feels about you anytime and anywhere.
- *how to* learn from your own life by interacting with God about your memories and your current experiences.
~~~

My friend Tony described his experience with reading an advanced copy of this book.

> *Until last year, I never thought Jesus could speak clearly to me. I assumed for most of my Christian life that He spoke through the Bible and even through other people but not directly or clearly to me.*
>
> *But when I read Lisa's dialogue with God I was amazed. Could one possibly have that intimate a relationship with the Lord? A year or two ago I would have rubbished the idea. Having opened myself up to the idea of hearing from Jesus, I now long for it. Who doesn't want that kind of intimacy with the Lord?*
>
> *Because of this book, I expected more, I expected a more intimate conversation with Jesus. I said, "Jesus if you can do this with Lisa, I'll take a chance and believe you will talk to me in the same way."*
>
> *When the book is published I will be recommending it to all my Christian friends, telling them "Jesus speaks to us. Don't believe me? Read this book."*

Early in the writing process, my writing coach, Marcy, asked, *"Isn't this really a book about prayer?"* Prayer can mean so many different things, and I don't want a negative association with that word to prevent someone from investigating this book. I define prayer as our honest, imperfect, and ongoing conversations with our Creator whom we choose to pursue a relationship with. Is this a workable definition for you? If so then I enthusiastically say, *"Yes. This is a book about prayer. Welcome. I am glad we are here together. Let's read this book as if you and I are visiting and God is there too, patiently smiling at you and waiting for you to invite Him to* join the conversation."

CHAPTER 1
The Road Map
Where We Are Headed and How We Are Traveling

Have you ever been alone and felt overwhelmed and paralyzed with stress, confusion or sadness? I compare it to driving down the highway, having one tire on the gravel shoulder, and then ending up in a ditch. In fact, many of my hardest moments of being bombarded with negative thoughts occurred when I was driving alone in the car.

What if you could get yourself back on track, clear-headed, relaxed, and grateful even when you feel lonely, anxious, or triggered with painful memories? What if you could stay connected to God even when you feel ashamed or angry and actually hear God's perspective on your situation? What if you could rest assured that God can handle all that and be happy to stick with you?

t if when a negative thought pops in your head you decide, *"Oh, I am not going there"* and you just keep driving down the road? What if this *"road"* isn't leading you to work or the gas station but on an adventure? On this road trip, you are not sure what might be around the bend, but you are just glad to be out there. You feel resilient, hopeful, and confident that you and God can handle anything together.

I can pose these scenarios because I have experienced them. I have learned how to stay on the road, avoiding unnecessary obstacles. I have also learned how to more quickly get myself out of the ditch when I feel despair and negativity.

Do you ever get tired of reading books or listening to podcasts on *"how to improve"* and wish that instead you could simply watch the author live? Sure, you are going to chart your own course and you wouldn't want to handle life the exact same way anyone else does, but wouldn't it be great if you could get some new ideas to fuel your unique responses to the hard stuff of life?

I invite you to hang out with me and see a bit of how I have lived through the tougher times, with God involved through them. Envision yourself hopping in the back seat of my car and joining me for a stretch of highway on the road trip. Eavesdrop on my conversations with God! I am honest about my feelings, questions, disappointments, and the toll that it takes on my body and relationships.

I hope when I describe my feelings that you remember feeling something similar.

I hope when I ask God questions that you remember some questions you have asked.

I hope when I describe feeling stress in my body or exhaustion that you can relate to those feelings.

I hope when I describe my disappointments that you remember feeling disappointed.

Since I want you to stay in the car with me, I will keep the descriptions of my troubles mild and minimal. It is important to me that you are not overwhelmed or distracted by the details of my circumstances. I remember when I was searching for help, many resources were peppered with tmi.[1] While reading other peoples' trauma stories, I often felt more despondent instead of hopeful and empowered to overcome.

My conversations continue past my laments to reveal God meeting me in every situation.

I hope when God shares His perspective with me, you anticipate that reframes are always possible.

I hope when God validates me, you anticipate God will validate you.

I hope when God comforts me, you anticipate God will comfort you.

I hope when I bounce back with joy and renewed purpose, you anticipate that recovery is possible.

Our brains have amazing power to shift and form new and powerful thoughts when we hear someone else's story. I just love how God created us!

~~~

Speaking of stories, my daughter Sophia made a brilliant discovery. Watching reruns of The Andy Griffith Show has a lot of benefits without the unwanted side-effects of many contemporary shows, which desensitize us to violence, disrespect, and entitlement. According to Sophia:

> *"Andy always finds a way of comically showing people their faults without violence or shame so they just feel silly for not noticing their own flaws. He is the sheriff, yet he doesn't even*

1. Too much information.
~~~

carry a gun. He stays aware of people's feelings and actively makes sure everyone still feels okay about themselves. If someone does have a flaw, he helps them as much as possible so they don't feel like it is a big deal."

My husband and I enjoyed watching some episodes with her and seeing it through her eyes of appreciation. I was being mentored in how to navigate the trials of life while remaining kind to others, no matter how troublesome the relationships seemed. I wonder what would happen if we all watched *Andy Griffith* for a month? What habits would we pick up from him?

Although I am not *yet* as witty as Andy, I hope that as you hang out with me, you will pick up some ideas on navigating the trials of life while keeping it real with God. So just like Andy and the community in Mayberry, perhaps my stories will provide you with a new way of looking at God, yourself, and others that will solve problems without false guilt, toxic shame, or heavy-handedness.

~~~

The remainder of this chapter has recommendations for how to approach the book and reflect on it. It also contains brief stories about my background.

Format

Conversations in this book are formatted like a script. "*L*" indicates me, Lisa. "*G*" indicates God. I understand God in three persons: God the Father, Jesus the Son, and Holy Spirit. God is my Daddy in Heaven in a way that transcends even our best experiences or imaginations of a loving Daddy. I passionately believe that God created males and females equally valuable and that God embodies all the best qualities of male and female but is not constrained to either one. Sometimes I refer to God using
~~~

masculine pronouns. I hope that isn't a hindrance. Since Jesus the Son walked this earth then crushed death, He is with me like a friend and simultaneously working powerfully for my greatest good with all the best resources. Holy Spirit helps me experience Jesus as if He is right next to me telling me what is true. What a team!

Chapters two through eight consist of my conversations with God. After each conversation or group of conversations, I reflect on what I learn. While I have devoted the past thirty-four years to cultivating my relationship with God, most of what I share occurred over a four-year period when I felt most desperate for intimacy and help from God.

The conversations are organized by what I learned, obstacles I removed, and struggles I overcame. The following is a list of chapter titles with accompanying lessons for each. Just for fun, many of the titles are from songs that I sensed God inviting me to sing:

Chapter 2—Something in the Way She Moves: From Paralyzed to Deliberate

Choose to trust Jesus, the real Jesus, without distortions, accepting that I will spend the rest of my life discovering who He really is and what He is really like..

Chapter 3—When God says, "After you": From Hidden to Authentic

Take care of myself because my life is valuable. My mental health is my most valuable asset.

Chapter 4—I Can See Clearly Now: From Confused to Confident

Trust my instinct, re-establish and discover new aspects to my identity.

Chapter 5—Can't Stop the Feeling: From Ambivalent to Alive

Embrace emotions, and choose what I do with them.

Chapter 6—I Have to Say I Love You in a Song: From Prideful to Teachable

Be a lifelong student in the school of love, willing to give up attitudes and methods that are not working and seeking to learn what is needed.

Chapter 7—Ain't Too Proud to Beg: From Self-Sufficient to Vulnerable

Ask for help from God, unafraid of being vulnerable with God.

Chapter 8—Freeway of Love: From Protective to Adventurous

Build up a memory bank of God's dynamic, reciprocal presence in my life.

When I needed extra support dialoguing with God about painful situations, I worked with a coach who took notes while I interacted with God so I could focus on what I was feeling and hearing. I believe it is crucial to be selective and cautious when working with a listening coach. With all the available methods, techniques, and training in praying for others, we can become over-reliant on others to do our work. Likewise, coaches who assert too much power, knowledge or act with a sense of superiority can detract others from establishing their own connections with God. Unfortunately, I speak from more experience than I wish I had on both sides of these equations. However, this has driven me to learn how to go to God first and to do only what is needed to support others until they themselves can do the same.

~~~
~~~

How to approach the book

Following are several suggestions on how to approach this book:

- Stay curious instead of judgmental
- Name the shame
- Give your brain permission to refrain from determining the details of my distress
- Give your brain permission to refrain from creating a timeline of events and conversations
- Give your brain permission to use all of its parts
- Give your heart permission to feel
- Give your body permission to relax
- Pay attention to cues that your mind, heart, and body are inviting you to respond to
- Determine when *you* want to respond
- Record your responses in a journal
- Remember that God is with *you*, wanting to hear your heart
- View my conversations as descriptive, not prescriptive
- Ask God questions
- Take your time
- Take it personally

Stay curious instead of judgmental

This applies towards yourself, me, and all the other Christians you have ever known. This can be a hard discipline to practice. Curiosity helps keep our minds open to having a new thought—perhaps a thought that could only come from God. It helped me to make this hard shift by stopping and saying out loud, "*I wonder...*" and determining how to finish the sentence when inside I was saying, "*I know...*" For example, when I started to think, "*I know that person is just trying to justify herself at my expense*" I would say, "*I wonder what they want and need right now. I wonder what I can and cannot provide.*"

Name the shame

Shame whispers, *"I could never really be intimate with God or feel loved,"* but it is usually camouflaged with other sophisticated statements. For example, we might say we need to acquire more knowledge about God or the Bible before we can have a deeper relationship. Now that I can identify when I feel shame, I sort shameful thoughts and feelings into three categories: toxic shame, reparable shame, and realistic shame.

Toxic shame says something like, *"There is something wrong with me. I can't talk and listen to God for real. Others might be able to have this, but I never will. I am disqualified because of my ____________ (e.g. irreparable history, weakness, immaturity…)"*

I learned that honesty with God yields great results. Even when I felt blocked from God, I told Him about my thoughts, feelings, and doubts. It helped to talk out loud and hear myself. For example, *"God, I feel like giving up on us. I am afraid if I try talking and listening to you, nothing will happen, and I will feel even more alone. I am afraid that I am too messed up to ever have an intimate relationship with you. I feel left out from what others seem to have, and I am too weary to put myself out there again. I am not sure you will come through for me, but could you show me that I qualify just as much as anyone else in being able to experience that you are with me?"*

Reparable shame says, *"I messed up, and I receive this gentle alert so I can see how I want to change."* I like to be straight with myself and God and say something like, *"I have made some mistakes. I want to learn from them and adapt. God will you forgive me? I receive your forgiveness. I forgive myself. Help me act like my best, true self. Help me identify any repairs that I am responsible for and follow through to make those repairs. I acknowledge those who hurt me in this "mess up,"* and I forgive those who hurt me."

Realistic shame says, *"I don't measure up, and I accept the gift of being set free from the demand to never make a mistake."* It helps me to accept this fact and desire change. I felt so liberated once I learned that sin is not meeting God's standards and that no one can live up to them in this life. I began saying to God, *"I realize I am not _________ but I want to be. Can you please help me be more like you? Please help me to be ________."*

Give your brain permission to refrain from determining the details of my distress

The popularity of violent and horror-filled media offerings indicate how we are easily drawn to gory stories. Please consider filtering this part of your imagination, so you will not be distracted from seeing how God and I interact.

Give your brain permission to refrain from creating a timeline of events and conversations

Since I was learning many things at once and having conversations on different topics at the same time, it seemed best to organize chapters by the theme of what I was learning.

Give your brain permission to use all of its parts[2]

One part of our brain that is most concerned about our survival tends to overreact when we are trying something new, a little risky and transformative—even taking the risk of trusting God with our hearts. One of my coaching clients said her biggest takeaway from our twelve coaching sessions was the session when she wrote that part of her brain a letter saying, *"Thank you very much for ensuring my survival and for warning me that I am embarking on new territory. I will be fine. You can chill out now."*

2. Chapter nine contains more description of how I understand the right and left sides of my brain.

Give your heart permission to feel

Please consider this book as your permission slip to interact with God about your own similar feelings. This is easier said than done. Here are a few things that helped me. I listened to the story and sang the song, "*Tell your heart to beat again.*"[3] I embraced what Brene Brown says, "*We cannot selectively numb emotions. When we numb the painful emotions, we also numb the positive emotions.*"[4] I wailed and discovered that I survived. I discovered that Jesus stayed with me in my sadness and lightened my load.

Give your body permission to relax

A few deep breaths and taking care of your body so it is free of tension or pain will help your mind consider new thoughts.

Pay attention to cues that your mind, heart, and body are inviting you to respond to

Try to pause whenever something positive or negative impacts you. Perhaps you notice that you feel sad, angry, excited, or distracted. Maybe you want to search online for other information or check on social media. Perhaps you start to crave a certain food or a drink even if you are not hungry or thirsty. Maybe your analysis or criticism of my methods or beliefs is in overdrive. These could be signs that you are trying to protect your heart from the pain of identifying with me. These could all be cues that it is time to stop, set this book down, and reflect. Zoom in on your heart and the right side of your brain in these important micro-moments to identify what you are really wondering and feeling. Also notice if you are storing any pain or tension in a particular place in your body.

---

3. Gokey, Daniel. *Tell Your Heart to Beat Again*. YouTube. https://www.youtube.com/watch?v=eUHRDCYnFfg

4. Brown, Brene. *The Gifts of Imperfection: Let Go of Who You Think You're Supposed to Be and Embrace Who You Are*. Center City, MN: Hazelden, 2010.

Determine when *you* want to respond

I want you to sharpen this skill and trust yourself. If I gave you a series of questions to answer or exercises to do at the end of each chapter, I would prevent you from paying attention to your heart. Do you want to stop and reflect mid-paragraph? Go for it.

Record your responses in a journal

There are wonderful journaling exercises that I have benefitted from, but since I am promoting *real talk* with God, I invite you to try being real and raw with blank pages. You can always check out my resource list for ideas later, but I discovered that once I started creating something out of nothing (an empty sheet of paper), the words on my page were transformative.

Remember that God is with you, wanting to hear your heart

I believe God created each of us and is always with us, wanting to hear our hearts whether we believe or experience that as true or not. This is what kept me going through the darkest times. Can you employ the tiniest bit of belief that this is true *for you*, and then ask God to show you He is with you and wants to hear your heart?

View my conversations as descriptive, not prescriptive

Allow them to fuel your awareness of how God might be communicating with you, but don't try to extract a step-by-step, linear explanation of how to have a conversation.

Ask God questions

That's when the real transformation and fun began for me. God is so creative and in touch with our lives. I distinguish between two types of questions: those that clarify confusion and those that are more for the sake of relationship. Sometimes they merge. I like to jot my question down in a journal and let the answer unfold as days, weeks, and months follow. God has a much better memory than I do, and I love it when he remembers and answers the ones I don't record. (See Ask for the Ancient Paths in chapter seven.)

I love hearing the clients I coach asking God questions.[5] During one session with a client who wanted to experience the love of God in daily life, she asked Him, *"Could you please show me doing something fun with you?"* (This is the type of question that began for the sake of relationships.) She envisioned herself fishing with God. This triggered memories of how she experienced God's care and protection when fishing in the past. Not only did she enjoy peace and relaxation relishing these memories, she went fishing for the first time in years that same day. She created an action step in self-care consisting of casting a line for fifteen minutes a day.

Feel free to jot down the questions I ask to use as conversations starters. I wonder what questions you will come up with as your curiosity grows. Are there some ice breaker questions you could ask God just for fun?

Take Your Time

One of my clients said to make sure I tell my readers, *"This takes time and effort."* Consider this a transcontinental road trip not a jaunt across town.

A few specifics on responses that have worked for me

Remember these are not prescriptions just suggestions:

- Write out my dialogue with God.
- Cry with grief.
- Write and send a letter of appreciation or acknowledgement.
- Write and send a letter of apology.

---

5. To join an online small group that focuses on relational discipleship, listening to God and listening to each other, you may request to work with me as your facilitator at https://deeperwalkinternational.org/journey/ I coach clients in areas of physical, emotional, relational, spiritual health and leadership. Please email me at lisa@lisadodgepinkham.com if you are interested in coaching.

- Read one of my conversations out loud (this helps connect both sides of the brain).
- Read one of my conversations/stories to a trusted friend and notice how we feel and if we sense our minds shifting out of negativity.
- Move my body. I love to take a dance break to a favorite song, or walk while talking to God.[6]
- Sometimes I use the voice recorder on my phone to record my conversation when I am walking.
- When I participate in some form of a small group, we take time to be quiet together and listen to God on our own. Then we share with each other what we thought we heard.

A little more about me

"I want you in my life FOREVER—no more wavering back and forth," I silently told God during the middle of a church service, as December finals of my sophomore year in university approached. Just a few weeks prior, I resolved to return to church and figure out how to make sense of life and God. I wanted to know how to get all that I was supposed to out of both my education and Christmas.

I knew Christmas was a really big deal. But, despite my efforts to make and purchase the perfect gifts and to support meaningful family traditions, it always felt like I had yet to access the satisfaction of Christmas deep in my soul. After spending most Sunday mornings of my childhood at our small church in rural Maine and then wandering in and out of churches during my first year in university, I asked one of my best friends Lisa if I could go to church with her. She was an acquaintance in high school who

6. Here is my current favorite dance song for building joy and appreciating people: Timberlake, Justin. *"Can't Stop the Feeling."* YouTube. https://www.youtube.com/watch?v=ru0K8uYEZWw.

transferred to my university that autumn. The first day she drove to campus she said Jesus felt so close to her, she literally cleared off the passenger seat to honor Him with a physical place to sit. I still thank Jesus for escorting her back into my life so that I could ask her about church. Three Sundays after going to that church, I made that private request for God to be in my life forever, and He took me up on the offer.

Two months prior to that, I visited a different church with Lisa and listened to other college students talk about how God changes their lives. I remember thinking, *"I am so bummed I missed that boat. I will never have that."* (Noticing the toxic shame talking there? Why did I disqualify myself?)

When I first entered university I filled out a survey during orientation which led to a follow up visit from an older student to my dorm room. She asked me whether God or I was ruling on the throne of my life. I told her that I was on the throne. When she asked if I wanted to keep it that way or have God on the throne, I responded, *"I want God on the throne, but I am really busy with school and need to make the most of my education. I would probably need to change my major and do something less time consuming and demanding in order to have God be on the throne."* I spent my first year discovering that I really liked my major—exercise physiology, and my minors—dance and psychology. I didn't want to give them up for God. How liberating it was in my sophomore year when God seemed to say, *"Yes! Atta girl, Lisa! I designed you to be with me* as *you pursue your interests. Let's do this together!"*

For the next thirty years, I wholeheartedly embarked on the journey to love, understand, and serve God without hesitation or doubt that He and I were in each others' lives. I worked in ministry to college students, got married to an amazing follower of Jesus, went to seminary, raised two incredible daughters, and founded and directed my own dance school. I taught homeschool classes for twelve years and spoke and wrote about the love of God with my children, their friends, in small groups, and at churches.

What happened?

About three years ago, however, I crashed into a roadblock that took me down and out. I felt sad and exhausted, like I was carrying a wet wool blanket over my shoulders. Grief sometimes overtook me to the point where, rather than shedding a few tears, I sobbed, wailed, and felt deep pain in my gut. I questioned the value and meaning of my life, wondering if I could ever get back on track to a purposeful existence. My anxiety increased. Nothing that previously worked was effective.

If we define abuse as the misuse of power, there were several ways that I experienced this, spiritually and relationally. Some of the relationships and spiritual communities I was in kept triggering the message that I was inferior. It was especially traumatic to encounter similar abuses from those I sought support from.

The dark night of the soul is an apt description that is rarely used these days, but we could certainly call it that. I remember lying on my bed unable to sleep in the middle of the night saying, *"God, everything I thought was essential to my relationship with you has been ripped out from under me. Even the sacred, secret places I had with you have been defiled. I try to read favorite Bible verses, sing favorite songs that help me connect with you, or take communion. Before I know it, though, I am triggered by painful memories. I know you are there under all this mess. Please show me where you are. Show me how to be with you with nothing between us and how to travel light and simply on this journey with you."*

In keeping with my commitments not to share too many details and to take responsibility for myself, I can explain a few more things. As my sense of powerlessness and vulnerability increased in conjunction with the greater intensity of life challenges, I regressed into an overreliance on external authorities, which I needed to overcome. Unfortunately, I have also witnessed this in other people whom I once viewed as strong, capable, and confident, so I also needed to break away from that crowd.

I stopped suppressing my emotions and allowing others to dismiss them. Once I determined to live from my heart no matter what, I faced a steep learning curve on how to respond to the sadness, despair, anger, fear, and disgust that was surfacing.

I worked hard to strengthen my skills in speaking up. Clarifying misunderstandings, respectfully declining from doing something I didn't want to do, refusing to do things I was opposed to, and advocating for those who could not speak for themselves became high priorities.

These self-initiated changes disrupted the status quo and brought challenges to my existing relationships. I learned how to handle others' responses to these changes. This was messy but worth it!

Bouncing back

When I act like my best, true self, I am tenacious, and I don't give up. So, I diligently sought after new environments and tools that I could employ for healthy functioning in daily life. My highest priority was to restore and deepen my relationship with God and to be more real with Him.

My big question: What does real talk with God look like?

If a personal relationship with a personal God is what distinguishes Christianity from other spiritual beliefs, then why does prayer usually seem like a monologue? It seems like either we do all the talking or we think God does.

What did it look like when I did all the talking? Sometimes I only asked Him for help or money, or I only thanked Him. Then there were the times of mostly complaining. At least that was honest and we can find plenty of examples of that in the Bible! Reciting prayers others have spoken for centuries and turning Bible verses into prayers have been very useful when I just couldn't, or didn't want to, come up with my own words. But that's all talking and no listening.

On the other hand, why do we think God should do all the talking? When I took classes on how to listen to God during prayer, I kept company with those who sensed God speaking in lengthy discourses. God seemed to be saying just what we needed to hear, but I was not convinced this characterized an intimate two-way relationship.

In ancient times, as described in the Old Testament, people knew about God but didn't yet grasp that he was going to be transported to earth as a completely dependent human baby, enduring all the human growing pains of moving from childhood to adulthood in a hostile environment. It is recorded that *"God spoke with Moses face-to-face as neighbors speak to one another"* (Exodus 33:11, The Message).

I believe that the distinguishing factor of Christianity is that we can know and be known by a personal God who created us, walked in our shoes (well, Jesus likely walked in sandals), and proceeded to do what only He could do. He became the only God who died, beat death, and returned to life as a completely powerful and compassionate God. I am convinced that since we are on this New Testament side of history, then I ought to be able to have more than just a neighborly conversation with my Creator. As previously mentioned, I think it should feel like I am on a road trip with God. He and I are cruising on a grand adventure—talking and listening, silently taking in all the new sights, enduring stormy weather, and reveling in the sun when it shines.

~~~

As you head into the rest of the book, consider Tony's example of responding to the advanced draft of the book. He demonstrated an inner drive and belief that propelled him to chart his own course in dialoguing with God. I hope his approach to the book will inspire and motivate you.

> *I am on a week's retreat in a cell at a Monastery near where I live. I come here around this time every year to wait on the Lord and try and discern what He might want to say to me. Sometimes I get something, and sometimes I just rest. It is always a good time even if it takes a little getting used to at first.*
>
> *I have been experimenting with Immanuel Journaling*[7] *for the last while and it has had an impact on me to a degree. Jesus is nearer, and I feel my relationship with Him is stronger.*
>
> *On the second night of my retreat, I woke at 4:00 a.m. wide awake. I asked Jesus what He wanted me to do. He said, "read Lisa's book." I got up and read half of the book. I laughed and I cried. Most of the time I said, "Wow! I want this, I want this." Then I asked myself, "Does Lisa have a special gift of hearing the Lord or could this be for everyone? Who wouldn't want to hear the beautiful voice of their creator talking to them in such a loving, caring way?"*

---

7. Wilder, James, Anna Kang, John Loppnow, and Sungshim Loppnow. *Joyful Journey*. East Peoria, Ill.: Shepherd's House, 2015.
~~~

When I got up the following day I finished the book (wished it went on and on). When I put it down, I prayed and asked the Lord to talk to me just like that.

I quieted myself for a time, and I thanked Jesus for blessings He has given me, took up my pen, and waited. Jesus spoke to me in an intimate way like never before, again and again...

I have had several conversations with Jesus. I dared to do what Lisa has done. I asked Him to go back to places in my past and meet me there. There were tears and laughter all in great safety. There was release and even singing. This very day I have seven pages of intimate dialogue with Jesus in my journal.

~~~

As you read my conversations with God in chapters two through eight, some questions might arise. Or perhaps you will feel stuck in a strong reaction and unable to move forward authentically. Feel free to flip ahead to chapter nine and peruse my responses to questions. I hope this information will empower you to return to the conversations.

Now that you have looked at the overall road map of our journey, I invite you to relax and join me as I recount personal stories and conversations with God that have truly healed my mind and put me back in the driver's seat on a most adventurous road trip through life.
~~~

CHAPTER 2

Something in the Way She Moves

Paralyzed to Deliberate

Deliberate: carefully weighed or considered; studied; intentional, leisurely and steady in movement or action; slow and even; unhurried.[1]

As I was emerging from my funk of insecurity and purposelessness, I realized that I needed to re-establish my ability to bring myself to God.

Bringing myself to God without relying on others to help me get to Him is vitally important. One afternoon, while in the midst

1. dictionary.com

of this readjustment, I set aside some time to *have it out* with myself and God.

~~~

The Glory Sheet

L: I don't care how long I have to walk and talk with you. I am determined that I am going to connect with you on my own, independent from a class and without someone prompting or coaching me. Let's do this. Just you and me, God. Now that I have walked, and sung, and said the Lord's Prayer for the past half hour, my body and mind feels relaxed. I expect to sit still in this beautiful spot in the woods and look at the pond until I see you more clearly. The residual racing thoughts should quiet when I complete these relaxation exercises. Okay. Let's try this—What memory do you want me to appreciate?

G: Remember when you were in your mid-twenties and you returned to Acadia and hiked the Bubble Rock Trail? Upon reaching the summit, you stretched out in the sun, munched on your trail mix, and stared at the two mountains named Bubble Rock.

L: Yes, what a beautiful day and refreshing getaway after a very busy season.

G: Your friend took a photo of you, and you kept it at your desk for years.

L: Between my pink shorts, teal shirt, and the blues and greens of the mountains, trees, and skies—it was a vibrant photo. Every time I looked at it, I felt more alive with joy and at the same time drawn to be at peace. I wrote a quote under the photo about how the carpenter's son (Jesus) went away to quiet places to be with you. Where were you then?
~~~

G: Can you sense me already stretched out on the rock inviting you to join me for rest and enjoyment of our creation?

L: Yes, that makes sense that you were making *"me lie down in green pastures"* and restoring *"my soul"* (Psalm 23, NRSV).

G: I am glad you see who I am, what I am like, and that I want to care for you.

L: What are you doing now?

G: I am here, inviting you to rest and enjoy my creation again. When you set out for your walk, you had no idea you would find this secluded spot in the woods in the middle of a city, which you have always found too busy and crowded.

L: You led me beside these *"still waters"* (Psalm 23, NRSV). Where are you now?

G: I am behind you, serving as your back rest so you can see the pond, the trees, and the birds and so you can relax on this rock.

L: It seems like you are acting like a sheet that is taut and utterly reliable for me to rest back on. I feel secure and comfortable. I can't see you, but I sense you—a shimmering white sheet that is both soft and firm enough to lean into. I will remember this as the glory sheet.

G: I am glad you persisted in being with me today.

The next morning, my fifty-first birthday began when I met a friend at a coffee shop. On display were paintings depicting scenes from the book Solomon's Song of Songs in the Bible. Captivated by one particular painting, I imagined placing myself in it. A woman dressed as a bride placed her hands on her heart as she leaned back into Jesus—the groom whose hands were on her hands.

L: God, you aren't just a sheet behind me, you are Jesus, a person, the Groom.

G: And you are my beautiful bride.

L: You are my Groom? What timing to see this today after yesterday.

G: Every step you take toward me on this journey will reveal more of who I really am in this world, and who I want to be for you.

L: I want to keep moving toward you. I would love to find a way to purchase that painting and remember this.

Later that day, I opened up a birthday card from my parents with a check for the exact amount of the painting. I immediately thanked God for orchestrating the timing and arranged to purchase the painting from the artist.

L: Thank you, God, for walking with me step by step as I continue opening my heart up to you more and more. Thank you for being in sync not only with what I need, but what I want. I feel so noticed, validated, and desired, especially on my birthday.

I placed the painting in my bedroom so I could begin each day with a visible reminder of God's personal love and involvement in my life. These memories of my walk, the glory sheet, seeing the painting, and then purchasing the painting became the foundation from which other memories would be added. Hanging the painting was like creating a cairn, the piles of stones used to mark hiking trails. Every time I saw it, I thought about how God is looking out for me. It reminded me of how God often instructed the Israelites to put a pile of stones to mark a place where He rescued or guided them. Whenever anyone came across the stones, God's loving investment in people's lives would be projected as the story was retold. There are many accounts of this recorded in the Old Testament, and in one story, Samuel named the stone "Ebenezer; for he said, thus far the Lord has helped us" (1 Samuel 7:12, NRSV).

If we were taking a trip through my brain, I imagine that we would be creating new cairns to lay out the story of God's faithfulness so that the next time I hiked that path, I could see each cairn and remember what God had already done for me. I needed that when I was having a really tough day...

Remember the Glory Sheet, Access Me Yourself

L: I am just beginning to grasp how vastly isolated and rejected I feel. What a toll it has taken on me. It is worse than I thought. What do you want me to remember, God?

G: Remember when you went on that walk and kept asking me to help you, asking all by yourself? You experienced me as the glory sheet that you could lean back into?

L: Yes, I felt strong, safe, and reassured that you had my back. The next day, I saw the painting of the bride leaning back into your arms. That painting reminds me of how I spent a year reading Song of Songs each day, yearning to give and receive a purer love. It is so confusing right now. Sometimes, I can't even read that part of the Bible without being overcome by the stream of negative memories associated with it.

G: I am sorry that it is confusing. The words of the Bible are meant to be life-giving, but people make their own choices about how they use them. You are free to choose as well. In this very moment, you can choose what part of these memories you want to focus on.

L: Can I choose? Really? I don't choose to be triggered. Often, I am minding my own business, and memories invade me unannounced and uninvited.

G: Lisa, I know how painful this is for you. You can choose how to respond when you are triggered. You can also consider it from my perspective.

L: It is inconceivable that I can choose and respond differently. Let's give this a shot. Yes, please show me your perspective.

G: As hard as that season was, the spiritual alienation was not without purpose. I was there with you, walking beside you. That process led you to realize what you don't want or need so you would ask for the *real deal* with me.

L: This resonates with me on a certain level, but at the same time, there is a lot of mess, division, and disillusionment with the most important relationships in my life.

G: Is there a way you can acknowledge where you are in this moment of anguish and rejection without it overshadowing all that you have learned and are learning? Can you still lean back and rest on the glory sheet, on me?

L: It's reassuring, but obscure. You are still behind me and ungraspable, although I am leaning on you. I want to see your face, Jesus. I need more of you—more connection. I need to see that you want to be with me. That you are happy to be with me. That you accept me. Could you please give me a new way to experience your acceptance?

G: I am so glad to hear and see you opening your heart to me. I want this intimacy with you, too. I will answer the desires of your heart to feel accepted by me and deeply connected. Shall we move forward together?

L: Yes.

Decades ago, I remember hearing someone say, "God is a gentleman. He doesn't push or assert. Instead, God lets us choose." I am beginning to re-learn this truth and frame it in today's language; God is a coach. He waits for us to ask for help, asks great questions, offers invitations, and waits for our consent. It is vitally important that I choose to say "Yes" to God.

Sing a New Song to the Lord and Dance to It

L: Please, I need you. Please show me how to experience your acceptance. What obstacles are blocking me from seeing your face?

G: I am here.

L: I've gotten so confused with what is real and what is counterfeit in my relationship with you. Have I thrown the baby out with the bathwater of religion? If I have, I am so sorry.

G: No worries. Let's figure this out together. What do you need from me right now?

L: I am afraid to trust you. I need trust. I guess that means I need faith. Wow, that feels hard to admit, since I am supposed to have had it for over thirty years. I realize how afraid I am because I couldn't see how far off track we had gone from you. It has caused so much pain and regret. I need you most of all, but I am afraid of losing you again. After decades of pursuit, I thought I had arrived in this most holy, most sacred, most secret place with you...Now that very place has been invaded and defiled. I am afraid to trust you again because what if I make the same mistake? What if I can't separate you from the counterfeit? What if I am triggered and paralyzed by painful memories every time I try to connect with you?

G: I have new things for you, Lisa—really genuine, new things.

L: I am remembering the hymn *"Sing a New Song to the Lord."* I loved playing that on the piano and singing it. The sounds are deep and rich, and the melody reminds me of ocean waves. What is my new song?

G: Remember the Take 6 song *"Trust in Me Because I Love You"*?

L: Yes, that is a fun and funky song.

G: Do you want to sing it and free dance with me to it?

L: [giggling] Yes, I'll try.

G: How do you feel now?

L: Oh, things don't seem as painful. I just feel sad and angry. I should not have been squashed and invalidated. People should not misuse their power that way.

G: I agree. I feel sad and angry about that too. Do you want to go back and rest on the glory sheet?

L: Actually, I don't think that is what I need right now. I am not sure what is going on with me. Could you help me figure myself out? What do you want me to know about this?

G: Can you hear me singing another new song to you? It is a Michael Card song, *"...Show me your face, let me hear your voice, arise my love, arise and come to me."*

L: That's from Song of Songs.

G: How does it feel now thinking about Song of Songs?

L: Real and desirable—legit. You really want to see me and hear me, don't you?

G: Oh, yes. Do you want to see my face and hear my voice, Lisa?

L: Yes, but not like before where you seemed to pop in unannounced and indistinct.

G: Yeah, that doesn't sound like me. I love you enough that I want you to choose me. I am not going to pop up like magic. You will see the real me when you choose to come to me and invite me to come to you.

L: I get to choose and say "*Yes*" to you? I do choose. I know I have relied too much on others to help me make decisions. What does it mean to choose you?

G: Remember when I spoke to your husband when you were dating? You were both silently praying to me and asking if you could begin talking about and praying about marriage? I told him he could choose to marry you.

L: Oh, yes, he was so excited. He told me it was the first time he really heard your voice. It dissolved the pressure he felt to get it right in finding the one person on the planet you predetermined to be his wife. You invited him to think and feel with his whole heart and his whole brain.

G: I loved lightening his load and seeing his joy.

L: You give us the ability to choose. I do choose you. I do want to see your face. [Giggling] Now I sense you laughing and smiling, and it is different than how I used to experience your presence. Now, I am envisioning another painting in our home. The one of Jesus dancing with his bride. I am no longer leaning back onto you. I am the bride dancing with you face-to-face.

The following reflection occurred over many conversations and over several weeks. Sometimes, I was alone, and other times, I was with another person or in a small group where we were alternating between interacting with God about our memories and then describing the experience to each other. The best part was that I continued this authentic conversation even as I facilitated small groups and coached others on how to do this. Truly, the fact that

I can serve as a leader and teacher authentically, without burning out, has been most satisfying.

In Over My Head

L: I am not even sure how I feel right now, maybe numb. Maybe I don't want to acknowledge my pain and feelings. Shut down. That's it. But I don't want to stay here. I want to learn how to remember and listen and talk with you. Can you remind me of a time when I was peaceful and joyful, without pain and in awe of your creation?

G: Remember when you were seven years old and you spent the summer at the newly purchased cottage on the lake?

L: Yes, I loved being there.

G: One Saturday morning, your dad told you to climb on his back and wrap your arms around his neck, and he would swim you from the cottage dock to the neighbor's little beach.

L: Yes, I see myself happily chattering away while he is swimming, doing all the work.

G: How did you feel?

L: I felt strong, safe, and excited to try this new adventure. My body quivered with excitement and yet I kept it still so I could hold tight and stay on dad's back. It never occurred to me to be afraid even though I could not yet swim over my head. The sun sparkled on the water and twinkled all around me. I heard motorboats buzzing around, children playing, birds singing, and water splashing. What a delightful memory.

G: Do you wonder why I reminded you of this today?

L: Yes, why?

G: Perhaps you feel like you are in over your head with certain situations in your life, but I have you as long as you keep your arms around my neck and hold on tight.

L: This just makes me laugh. I certainly am in over my head, but I am drawn to your invitation to hold on tight to you and see you take me to a place that I could not arrive at on my own.

G: Let's go!

What About Jesus?

L: I am really curious. Since you are God in three persons, I am wondering where Jesus was and what He was doing when I was swimming on my Papa's back.

G: I was sailing around you in a sunfish sailboat with a red, white, and blue sail.

L: I envision you smiling, laughing, and enjoying watching us swim.

G: I lived on this earth, died, and rose again, defeating death so you could have this relationship with your Papa in Heaven.

L: Thank you. Thank you so much.

G: My pleasure.

Doing the Impossible

L: I am having fun with this. What about you, Holy Spirit? Where were you that day? Help me understand your unique role. Where are you? What are you doing in this scenario?

G: I am underneath you and your dad, walking along the bottom of the lake.

L: That's impossible.

G: Yes, that's my specialty.

L: I want to do that.

G: Come try it.

L: You are moving at a completely different rhythm than I am. With sure and steady footing, each step is deliberate, intentional, and firmly planted.

G: Yes, and I am unaffected by the noise and waves and activity above me.

L: When I feel the need to navigate life differently than everything around me, I will join you here under the water and learn your way of walking.

G: You are always welcome here and will join me in doing the impossible.

L: This reminds me of the unforced rhythms of grace that you, Jesus, spoke of:

> *"Are you tired? Worn out? Burned out on religion? Come to me. Get away with me and you'll recover your life. I'll show you how to take a real rest. Walk with me and work with me—watch how I do it. Learn the unforced rhythms of grace. I won't lay anything heavy or ill-fitting on you. Keep company with me, and you'll learn to live freely and lightly" (Matthew 11:28-30, MSG).*

The phrase "unforced rhythms of grace" began to ring in my head whenever I sensed tension and anxiety mounting in my body. Neck pain or chest tightness alerted me that I was not breathing fully. As I consciously relaxed my body and practiced my deep breathing, I imagined walking under the water with Holy Spirit, affirming that I wanted to move at Holy Spirit's pace, not my own. This often meant that I paid more attention to my internal thoughts and feelings and waited before speaking and acting. Thankfully, I had developed these habits well enough so that when I was paralyzed by a toxic conversation, I knew what to do and whom to turn to. The outcome was life-altering.

Acadia, Trust and Giggling

L: I just finished this really difficult phone call. Now I feel shaken and so vulnerable. It seems like the only bodily sensation I can identify is my nose. I can still smell. How bizarre to feel so disconnected from my body! Something in me needs to be stronger. I know I will be strengthened if I can rest in that secret place with you, with no interference. Could you please remind me of something to appreciate today?

G: Remember the hike you went on with your husband and daughter in Acadia National Park? I know how the Precipice is one of your favorite hikes.

L: Yes, it was my first hike ever. I was fifteen. Then thirteen years later I brought my husband on it. Twenty-three years after that, my seventeen-year-old daughter joined us. I felt so proud that I could still traverse those rock faces with iron rails. I felt tenaciously joyful sliding along the narrow paths, hugging the granite and looking out over the ocean. We giggled as we acted like our typical, always-dancing selves—extending our legs onto the iron hand rails with pointed toes as if they were our ballet barres. My husband acted as his true self, too, enjoying the hike and capturing photos of us on his cell phone. Even though I was battling a cold, I was determined that I would not miss out on this precious opportunity. I found an inner strength to not only persevere but also to thoroughly enjoy myself.

G: I enjoyed being on that adventure with you. Could you tell where I was?

L: It seemed like you were always just a little bit ahead of us, joking and laughing, saying, *"Come on, just a little bit farther. I can't wait for you to see this next view or to watch you overcome this next climbing challenge."*

L: It feels really important to me that this was such a positive, happy memory because my other daughter wasn't with us. When we went on a camping trip to the beach earlier that summer, I fought to overcome the idea that there was something wrong with me because she chose to be elsewhere. I guess I actually felt ashamed, like something in me was broken both because she wasn't with us and because I couldn't shake off my disappointment.

When we first headed to Maine for that vacation, I couldn't have imagined that I would go on this favorite hike and experience such joy without her being there. I also felt concerned that my other daughter would not fully enjoy herself without her sister being there. I know it is vitally important that our daughters make their own choices and find their ways of dealing with their own disappointments, but I felt so much sadness and fear that summer. What do you want me to know about that?

G: It is possible and important to experience all the good and pleasant emotions and moments I have given you in life, even when all your hopes and expectations are not fulfilled.

L: That feels true. I long for more of that. What do I need to get to that place where I can experience such contentment and trust?

G: Good question. What is your heart telling you?

L: *Sigh. * I just wish I could shake off my unbelief. That's it. Jesus, I feel afraid, vulnerable, and unprotected trying to trust you. My chest feels tight, like I can't breathe. There's something deep inside me that is cautious and holding me back. I want to trust you, but I am afraid I will get hurt. I want to learn how to enjoy moments again and create happy memories, no matter what circumstances surround me. But if I open my heart up to feel that joy, I also risk the pain of losing it.

G: I am with you to the extent that you want me to be, Lisa. I love you enough to keep my distance if that is what you need.

L: I remember when I first started experiencing your presence in a new way. It was as if you came into view as a bright, pulsating light. I felt so peaceful. The pulsing, rhythmic light soothed me like a baby wrapped in a parent's arms, hearing a lullaby. Even when I was praying with others, especially the Lord's Prayer, we would talk about how peaceful we felt. I never talked about the pulsating light with them because I didn't want to influence their own sacred experiences with you. Yet, somehow I sensed we were all experiencing your nearness in our own special way.

G: Yes, I remember that, too.

L: One time, as I was enjoying the pulsating light of your presence, it suddenly went away. The light turned into darkness, and the soothing rhythm abruptly stopped. I felt confused, afraid, and angered by the darkness. I was trying to trust you, but it was hard to get over losing feeling the warmth and light of your presence. I realize that I am afraid of trusting you and then having you disappear again.

G: I completely understand how you could see it that way. Thank you for telling me. Can you think of a time when you trusted someone and then they seemed to disappear?

L: Yes, once when I was a child, I remember feeling very alone in a situation where people I trusted had disappointed me. They weren't there for me the way I thought they would be. I remember standing alone saying, *"God, help me."* Even though I said the words, a part of me was just imitating what one of my friends told me she heard her older brother say one time when he was in trouble. But it seems like there was this other part of me that was venturing into new territory and really turning to you for help. I wasn't even sure I really knew you, but somehow I knew I needed to ask you for help.

G: I understand. You could have been doing both at the same time. You were learning and testing and trying to make sense during a confusing time.

L: Yes, it was confusing. I felt bewildered and betrayed. I wasn't used to feeling this way, and I wanted someone to tell me it would be okay and that I would be taken care of.

G: I know. Those are completely legitimate wants and needs. Can you tell where I was during that time?

L: Actually, I can now. When I decided to walk away from the situation, you came up beside me, put your left arm around my left shoulder, and held me tight as we walked to a place of rest. I could hear you saying, *"It is going to be alright, Lisa. You are all going to be alright."*

Once we got to a place of rest, I saw myself jumping into your arms, wrapping my arms around your neck, and giggling. I could feel your throat vibrating because you were giggling, too.

G: I am giggling, too, even now.

L: I feel hopeful, peaceful, and satisfied. I feel like I am being me. I can trust you now. Somehow, I know it is going to be okay.

G: Even as I am comforting you like a child, I am affirming you as an adult. You are so compassionate and caring. Even as a child, your heart of compassion and care for the people involved, including yourself, was developing. You have my caring heart in you. I am so proud of you.

L: This reminds me of one of my favorite children's books, *Where is Jesus?* I loved reading this book to my daughters. It depicts Jesus walking a child through some of the painful situations that arise in childhood and then asks the question, "*Where is Jesus?*" The reader opens a flap and reveals what Jesus is saying and doing in each situation. I picture myself now reading that same book to the little girl in me. Now I can see that you were there in the darkness and in every darkness.

G: Remember one of your favorite Psalms, 139? The one you told your daughters every night beginning when they were in your womb? Remember the words King David wrote about me, "*Even the darkness will not be dark to you; the night will shine like the day, for darkness is as light to you*"? (Psalm 139:12, NRSV)

L: Yes, I love that. You were walking beside me and holding me tight as I discovered the strength I had within me to choose to walk away to take care of myself. I told you earlier that something in me needs to be strengthened. Maybe the strength has always been there, I just need to acknowledge it.

G: What if I was prompting you to choose to take care of yourself and find inner strength you didn't know you had? What if I was inviting you to walk away and put yourself in a restful situation?

L: That makes sense to me now. I just sorted out a whole bunch of stuff in my mind and my heart. I believe I can trust you now. Especially when I feel your throat vibrating and hear you giggling with me.

G: Let's enjoy this together.

~~~

Although I inherited my mother's decorating style of covering every possible surface and wall with family photos, I adapted my own style once I began practicing this habit of remembering peaceful, joyful memories and interacting with God about them. Whenever I was in a beautiful moment worth remembering, I would take a photo, enlarge it, and hang it on the wall. A photo with a distant view of my daughter walking along the narrow rock path in Acadia, surrounded by natural beauty, hangs on the wall and invites me to sit still, breathe deep, and remember that moment, as well as the subsequent interactions with God.

Strategically placed photos invite me to stop and fill my mind with gratitude and connection to God. Perhaps they have subconsciously helped to keep my conversations with God fresh in my mind, enabling me to return to that topic and continue the dialogue with Him days, weeks, and months later.

Three-Legged Race

L: I feel utterly deflated. There has been a shift in one of the most precious relationships in my life, and the strain it is making on other relationships leaves me feeling like I have no one to turn to but you.

G: I am always here for you.

L: I have a five-hour flight, and I am just going to stare out the window and lean into you.

G: You and I can make a sacred, secret place anytime, anywhere.
~~~

L: Will you help me remember a time when I felt connected to you?

G: Remember when I showed you how I walked beside you when you were a little girl, you wrapped your arms around my neck, and felt my throat vibrating as I laughed out of the pure joy of being with you?

L: Yes.

G: My laughter didn't invalidate your sadness in any way. I shared that moment with you as we walked away together. BUT, my love for you and my delight in you and my pride in you was stronger than the grief.

L: I am beginning to grasp that we can actually hold seemingly contradictory feelings at the same time.

G: Yes, you are maturing in this just as you desired. I have heard your cries for help, and I am here with you, cheering you on as you step into the longings of your heart.

L: Even now I can feel your arm around my left shoulder and my right arm around your waist. Your strength and forward momentum is keeping me moving forward. But what about our legs?

G: Our legs? Remember the fun you had in three-legged races?

L: Yes, as a child, and even as an adult. I remember introducing the three-legged race to college students in Poland, and we had so much fun. We had to hold on tight with our arms to help us stay synced with our legs.

G: Can you envision your right leg and my left leg tied together to make one strong leg?

L: Yes, I need your leg tied to mine, serving as one. I need to know you are connected to me as I move forward and walk away from some things and toward other unknowns.

G: You got it.

L: I love how this childhood memory that used to be so distressing is now the memory I return to when I need comfort, strength, empowerment, and love. Why am I remembering this memory now?

G: What was your grief about then and what is your grief about today?

L: I am grieving about my loneliness and the seeming loss of connection with people I love.

G: Yes, I am sharing your sadness with you. Is there anything else?

L: Well, yes, there is more, and I am just accessing it deep in my heart now. Back then I felt grief and sadness because adults were not being adults in the way a child needed it. Today I am sensing that same type of grief.

G: I am sharing this grief with you. I invite you to keep holding tight to me, and we will move forward together.

L: I need to feel, to hear, to see you delight in me, and I need to trust you will stay with me. I need to experience the joy of being with you at a magnitude that supersedes the grief. I need to hear you giggling and feel our legs tied together as one.

The next four conversations progressed around the same theme for almost two years. I love envisioning what is happening in my brain as these new connections are made and difficult memories are reframed to become the inspiration that reframes the next difficult situation. I imagine a climbing ivy growing in length and breadth as more leaves expand from the vine.

Three Legs Are Better Than Four

L: I just read from Ephesians 3:20 in *The Message*: "*God can do anything; you know—far more than you could ever imagine or guess or request in your wildest dreams! He does it not by pushing us around but by working within us, his Spirit deeply and gently within us.*"

L: Your Spirit deeply and gently within me, Lord. That's what I want. I see myself holding on tight to you, Jesus, with our two legs tied together for a three-legged race.

G: What if the rhythm and pace we set for being tied together is better than if we were apart?

L: Three-legged races are fun and goofy, but not effective and efficient.

G: What if a three-legged race with me is both?

L: Really? You mean I am not slowing you down?

G: Right. And I am not slowing you down either.

L: Hmmm, have I thought that deep down?

G: Hmmm, take your time and consider it. In the meantime, what if each deliberate step we take together is more powerful, more glorious, more life-giving, and more impactful than if we were apart?

L: Three legs are better than four?

G: Each step you take releases more of my love and strength because we are tied together.

L: What a thought.

G: You know that verse you love from my book of *Romans*: "*The Spirit of God, who raised Jesus from the dead, lives in you. And just as God raised Christ Jesus from the dead, he will give life* *to your mortal bodies by this same Spirit living within you"* (Romans 8:11, NLT).

Apply here—to you and me in a three-legged marathon.

L: Go team!

Walking Away After 9/11

L: I am remembering a difficult memory. We had moved from New England to Northern Virginia and only been in the area a little over a year before 9/11. The girls were only five and almost three. I remember one night after snuggling with them in bed, reading stories, and praying with them, I stood in the doorway watching them sleep and wondered, *what if there is another attack and this is the last time I see them? There would be nothing I could do to prevent or control this. How do I live like this?* I felt so bewildered and full of hopeless despair, resignation, and fear. I reluctantly left the room they were sharing and walked down the long hall to our bedroom. I never shared those thoughts or feelings with you or anyone else. I had to shut my heart down some just to survive.

G: I know. I was with you, watching you with tender compassion as you worked so hard to silence those strong emotions and do the best you could to keep going. You created for your daughters a place of safety, fun, learning, creativity, and enjoyment for me to dwell in. You gave them stability and peace when they could have felt anxious and fearful.

L: I guess today is the day to bring these strong emotions and memories to you. I wonder why it is coming up today.

G: What do you think?

L: In 2001, I had to walk away from my little girls, leaving them in their bedrooms to sleep. Now they are grown women, independent and courageous and learning how capable and strong they are. How do I walk away from issues and problems that impact them, which are beyond my control, with trust instead of despair? How do I walk away appropriately yet still keep my heart engaged and readily available?

G: Is there a memory you have with me that you could appreciate right now?

L: Yes, I am remembering my three-legged walk with Jesus, which first began when I was walking away as a little girl.

G: See how I am connecting all these parts of your life? I have seen you and have been with you throughout your life.

L: Yes, I do see. I am glad that you *"are the same yesterday, today, and forever"* (Hebrews 13:8, NIV). I feel held by Jesus. He has me, and his left arm is holding my left shoulder. I feel the distinct rhythm of our three-legged walk. There is a jolt as our joined legs klunk. It is not as graceful or grounded as when I walk by myself. I want to get used to this and embrace it just as I embrace Jesus. I want to keep myself close to Him. I have to lean in and feel his left hand on my shoulder, pressing me against him for stability and unity.

How do I do this today, Jesus? How do I walk away and leave space for my daughters, my husband, others I love, and those I work with to deal with their stuff and live their lives? How do I walk away from situations beyond my control so that I can go back and have my own needed rest for the night? How do I find my own refreshment so I can appropriately engage when a new day dawns free of shame, full of forgiveness, accepting weakness, and appreciating the love we have for each other?

G: Those are excellent questions from a compassionate, loving heart.

L: Thank you. Jesus, I want to walk away with you to whatever new places, new people, new environments you have for me—wiser, more tender, more hopeful, less resigned and afraid. I see myself going back to my little girls and saying goodnight with an open heart. I will trust you to take care of them then and now. Please show me how you are taking care of each of them. Please remind me of a time when I knew that they knew you had them.

G: Remember when your youngest daughter stood in her bedroom after her open heart surgery and said, *"I feel God's love and safety-ness surrounding me through you and dad and all the people praying for me."* Remember when your family was on the missions trip to Brazil and your oldest daughter courageously took the initiative to determine to give up a toxic TV series, and then felt strong and free? Remember how your parents told their stories of feeling connected with me earlier in their lives? Remember how your husband felt when I surrounded him with my love while he was on his morning run? Remember the stories your friends have told of the joy and appreciation they have felt with you? Think of these things.

L: Yes, yes, I know this is what Paul told the Philippians to do: *"Fix your thoughts on what is true, and honorable, and right, and pure, and lovely, and admirable. Think about things that are excellent and worthy of praise"* (Philippians 4:8, NLT). I have been quoting that for decades. Ugh. This is really hard work that takes a lot of self-discipline. Please give me self-control and patience.

Every night our family has been asking you to give us the fruit of the Holy Spirit and listing them out: love, joy, peace, patience, kindness, goodness, faithfulness, gentleness and self-control (Galatians 5:22, NLT). I see now how much I really need self-control and patience.

G: Yes, it is deep work requiring you to choose which path your brain will take when despair tugs at you. Keep it up. I am proud of you.

Three-Legged Dance

L: I need you. Sometimes I feel like The Hydra in Greek mythology who just had her head sliced off. Now I know I can expect one, maybe two, to grow back in its place, but I hate feeling silenced and wounded as I wait for new growth. Can you please remind me of a time when my resilience deepened to help me get through this time without despairing?

G: Remember a few months ago when you were on that flight and I showed you that you were in a three-legged race with Jesus?

L: Yes, what a fun surprise that was. I am giggling just thinking about it. What do you want me to know about this, Lord?

G: I am really proud of you for coming to me with your whole heart as soon as you sat down on the plane. You didn't turn to a book, or work, or your phone, food, or despair. You pulled out your journal, looked out the window, thanked me for making the sky and earth so beautifully, then you brought me your pain.

L: I allowed myself to feel my pain and sadness with you. As a result, I experienced a new level of comfort.

G: I love how you keep remembering that and continue to interact with me afresh.

L: I resonate with the character of Peter in the Bible. When Jesus asked his twelve disciples if they would desert him, too, Peter said, "*Lord to whom shall we go? You have the words of eternal life. We have come to believe that you are the Holy One of God*" (John 6:68, NIV).

G: How does it feel to be in a three-legged race with Jesus?

L: I feel strong. I feel supported. His arm around my shoulder keeps my upper body supported. My waist to my toes are strong and supported, too.

G: When you have this strength in your body, it can support your heart.

L: My heart that feels so much pain?

G: Yes, with Jesus' body yoked to yours you will have the strength to live from your heart.

L: How does this memory connect with my life right now?

G: Just this morning you told me you couldn't bear the pain of being home alone, you couldn't bear the pain of trusting me with your daughter's hardships, you couldn't bear the insecurity of writing a book when you felt isolated.

L: I did tell you that, didn't I? Wow, I am glad I opened my heart up to you. You are answering my prayer, not by changing my circumstances but by being with me.

G: I want you to know that you are not slowing me down by being tied to me.

L: Really?

G: Yes, really. I also want you to know that I am not slowing you down either.

L: Oh wow. Do I really think that?

G: Do you?

L: That sounds so audacious, but yeah, I probably do think that sometimes. How awful. You have brought this up before and I didn't deal with it. I am so sorry.

G: No worries, I forgive you. You are just figuring *"us"* out as we go. That's what happens in every relationship.

L: You really are *"slow to anger and filled with unfailing love and faithfulness"* (Exodus 34:6, NLT).

G: I am glad you noticed. Instead of a three-legged race, what if we tried a three-legged dance?

L: Wait. What? I can relate to a three-legged race, and I can also relate to dancing the waltz or rhumba with you. Argh! I can't figure out how to dance with you with one leg tied to yours. The rhythm isn't right. There is no step that would work. Ugh. I can't relate to this. I have danced, and taught dance, all my life. This is unfamiliar. How can this be?

G: Do you want to continue on this adventure with me?

L: Yes.

G: Me, too. Enjoy letting me show you a new way to dance. I know the dance. I am holding you just tight enough. Your heart is open and you are strong. You can do this. We can even be graceful.

L: I am willing to try.

~~~

Three weeks after this conversation, a song I liked to dance to came on the radio. I began waltzing to it and imagining I was dancing with Jesus. I felt free, happy, and satisfied. I felt this nudge to imagine doing this as a three-legged dance with Jesus. Rather than getting
~~~

bogged down in how it could work without messing up our footing, I just kept dancing with the same abandonment. Somehow I was able to imagine my right hand in his left, my left hand forming a proper "V" below his shoulder and his left leg mirroring my right leg while having my right leg tied next to me.

Can you wrap your mind around that? Here lies the beauty of a life of faith—it is still beyond me as to how we do this, but I am enjoying it. His presence is enough.

Minimum of Four

G: Would you like to try a new dance?

L: Of course.

G: When you feel weak, needing to be strengthened, encouraged, and coached by me, you can always do the three-legged dance or three-legged race.

When you feel confident, excited, empowered, and adventurous, you can untie the belt binding our legs together and dance the ladies chain.

(In ladies' chain, with four dancers in a circle, two dancers move to the left and two dancers move to the right. Each dancer extends one hand forward, alternating right and left to grasp the hand of the dancer in front of them. They continually pass by one another.)

L: I am still connected with you, but different. This way I get to hold hands and look into the eyes of Daddy, Jesus, and Holy Spirit. I can see and appreciate each of you individually. I can hold hands and release hands, and I know I will come back to you.

G: Yes, when you feel weak and need me holding you tight, we can do the three-legged dance, or walk, or race. When you feel confident, empowered, and excited, you can untie the belt from our legs and dance with a little space between us. We are still united.

L: I feel supported and released simultaneously. This is freedom and connection at the same time.

G: Love looks like this.

L: I am beginning to see.

What better way to deliberately move toward freedom, adventure, and trust than to sell our home of sixteen years, declutter, downsize, visit family, house sit, take a road trip, and write a book for five months before moving into our next home? Traveling light is possible when I stick with my Constant Companion and "friend who sticks closer than a brother" (Proverbs 18:24, NIV).

You Know the Way

L: I feel lost, restless, and unable to settle. My well-staged house is calm, but I can't be still in it.

G: What can you remember and appreciate?

L: When you told your distressed disciples, "*You know the way.*"

G: Yes, I am the way, the truth, and the life.

L: Show me the way. I need help living this season of life. Preparing to leave the home where I raised my family, entrusting our house, money, and belongings to strangers, packing away the photos that help me get to my appreciation memories. How do I do this and stay connected to you?

G: What would it take for you to feel glad to be with every person you work with?

L: Joy.

Patience, especially in my tone of voice.
Kindness, thanking them for their work, accepting their limits.
Gentleness, being open to help.
Self-control, controlling my tone of voice *again*.

G: You got this. Let's do it together.

~~~

With the foundation of trust and desire re-established, and with hindrances and distorted thinking cleared, I was ready to choose to continue an authentic relationship with God. This prepared me for making the crucial, fundamental choice for another authentic relationship—the one with myself.
~~~

CHAPTER 3

When God says, "After you"

Hidden to Authentic

"My Life is valuable. My mental health is my most valuable asset." —Lisa Pinkham

Many of us have been taught phrases that shape how we prioritize our lives, such as: Jesus Others You (J.O.Y.); God Family Work; God Family Country. Imagine my surprise to sense Jesus saying, *"You First, Lisa."*

One day when I was in my mid-forties, I was considering some information that was very unsettling. I finally decided to stop swirling around my bedroom sorting and cleaning. I stopped, walked over to a chair, sat down and said:

L: God, I am thinking a lot about this situation. I am not sure what to think or how to feel about it. What do you think?

G: You go first.

This was a new situation for me. It was new for me to stop before my thoughts spun out of control and I was consumed with speculation and imagining the worst. It was new to ask God what He thought and how He felt. It was definitely new to sense God talking back. Hearing God tell me to go first—that was beyond unimaginable. It was a short conversation, but it stuck and whet my appetite for more.

The following conversations spanned three different seasons in my life. The first occurred before I started parenting preteens and while launching a dance ministry. The second series occurred after removing myself from toxic spiritual environments and as I began transitioning toward an empty nest and a new vocation. The third set of conversations occurred after I completed those transitions and became more attuned to the reality of aging. There is a fascinating progression of self-validation, self-care, appropriate self-sufficiency, interdependence with God, and interacting with God in the simple acts of daily life.

The first conversation occurred after having a dream that I would normally have dismissed as dark and disturbing. However, I was in the middle of a prayer course, which encouraged us to pay attention to the details of our dreams, investigating what they symbolized and contemplating what our minds needed to resolve. Oh, how important it was for me in those waking moments to engage with myself and God before rushing into the day, ruminating over my to-do list.

~~~
~~~

Nursing Myself Back to Life

The dream: I look down and discover that I am holding a baby in my arms. Initially, I am overflowing with love and tenderness—that beautiful dopamine-induced feeling of a precious life depending on me for attachment and care. Oh, how I loved being a mother to my newborn babies and immersing myself in providing a secure attachment for them.

The next time I look down, I notice this baby is grey. Why is she this color? I have never seen this before. Is this jaundice? No, this baby is indeed grey. The dreadful realization hits me… this baby is dead. However, before the flood of emotions hit me, I instinctively bring the baby to my chest. As she nurses, her cheeks become flushed with red. Her body melts into my arms and her little voice coos and gulps. I am literally nursing this baby back to life.

I wake with a start. Disgust and fear tempt me to absorb this as a soul-killing nightmare and to start my day with the brakes already on my heart. Instead, I choose to tune my heart to God first and determine to be an attentive student.

L: What do you want me to know about this dream, Lord? What does this grey baby turning rosy red represent?

G: Lisa, you are the grey baby. You, Lisa, are also the fast-acting, loving mom who instinctively brings the baby to her source of life and nourishment. You are nursing yourself back to life.

L: Me? Nursing myself back to life? Really?

G: I have given you everything you need. You can access all the resources I have given you. You can do this. Trust yourself. Trust Me in you. You have what it takes because you know I have what it takes. We will do this together, but it will happen when you believe you have what it takes to be life-giving and you choose to be life-giving for yourself.

L: I understand. I want this. This is a stretch for me. I am always helping others and chasing after help from someone else. I get it. I will learn how to nurse myself back to life. I see you holding me even as I am holding me.

G: I love how you are embracing this idea. I am so proud of you for learning from this dream instead of being disturbed and misinterpreting it as a nightmare. I am so proud of you for accessing your heart and mine.

During my twenties, when I was eager to please and learn from anyone and everyone who had been in a relationship with God longer than me, I often interpreted and applied Bible verses in a way that actually prevented me from taking care of myself rather than seeing them as words of life, intending to empower me to become my best, true self.

These habits deepened as the years went by, and I felt so much inner tension as I sought to inspire my daughters to learn to take good care of themselves even as I was struggling to figure that out for myself and authentically model that to them. This next interaction with God was crucial in freeing me from a distorted view of who Christ is and what He offers me.

Christ Moving in on My Weakness

L: I feel myself shutting down from you. I hear this Bible passage that was chosen for our reflection time in this Lectio Divina small group, and frankly, I am cringing. My body feels tense and anxious. My neck is tightening up, and I am not breathing fully or freely. I want to run out of the room. I don't want to sit here with this group and engage with this passage:

"Therefore, in order to keep me from becoming conceited, I was given a thorn in my flesh, a messenger of Satan, to torment me. Three times I pleaded with the Lord to take it away from me. But he said to me, 'My grace is sufficient for you, for my power is made perfect in weakness.' Therefore, I will boast all the more gladly about my weaknesses, so that Christ's power may rest on me. That is why, for Christ's sake, I delight in weaknesses, in insults, in hardships, in persecutions, in difficulties. For when I am weak, then I am strong." (2 Corinthians 12:7-10, NIV).

G: I am so glad you are honest with me. Please, tell me more.

L: Well, rather than work myself up about all the ways I have misapplied this verse and all the mandates I have heard from others, I think the best thing is for me to keep reflecting on different versions of this passage until something captures my attention.

G: Great idea. Take your time. I am with you, and I have all the time in the world.

L: I found something. I believe I can try to interact with this. *"My strength comes into its own in your weakness... It was a case of Christ moving in on my weakness"* (2 Corinthians 12:7-10, MSG).

Could you please show me what *"Christ moving in on my weakness"* really means?

G: You have this image in your mind of Jesus sitting on you, squashing you.

L: Oh, no. Really? Is that really what is in my heart? How awful. Please show me what it really means.

G: Envision yourself sitting on the right side of a smooth, grey bench. Jesus walks up and sits down at the far left end of the bench. You look at him with a smile and a *"Yes"* face that invites him to move closer. He slides along the bench, wraps his right arm around your shoulder and looks at your beautiful profile. He says, *"You got this, Lisa. You can do this. I am so proud of you, and I will always be here with you, coaching you."*

L: Wow. So you moving in on my weakness means you aren't squashing me or taking over? You are letting me be me. You are coaching me, and staying by my side. You are giving me courage and strength.

G: Absolutely, I understand what you are going through, and I am with you. I believe in you.

L: Talk about a reframe! Thank you.

G: I love doing that.

L: Yes, you even led the pastor through a reframe. Like many others, he thought the passage said: *"When I am weak, He is strong."* But what It actually says is: *"For when I am weak, then I am strong"* (2 Cor 12:10, NIV).

L: I feel so energized, confident, and empowered. I am so glad I stayed with you and the group this morning. I feel happy that I can share this good news with the group and hear their reflections.

G: I feel so happy seeing your whole group becoming all I intend for you to be as individuals and as a community.

The foundation stone of this memory was laid in September. The conversations on this topic continue to the present. In fact, the morning that I revised this chapter began with a strong feeling of overwhelm and fatigue, but I found the strength to move forward when God reminded me of this next conversation. I imagine this "cairn" as a tall stone tower.

Jesus and Me on the Bench

L: God, I feel so afraid, uncertain, and confused. My body feels paralyzed with weakness and insecurity. What do you want me to remember right now?

G: Remember Jesus moving in on your weakness on the bench with you?

L: Yes, absolutely. I love that memory. I can feel Jesus' arm across my back, firmly holding my right shoulder. I can hear him saying, "*You got this, Lisa. You can do this.*"

G: Good. Can you stay in that place and enjoy it? This can be your new secret place that you have been asking for.

L: Yes, but can you show me something beautiful? I love your creation and nature. What scenery surrounds us?

G: Actually, the bench is grey, and the scene around you is grey.

L: Really? This doesn't seem like you, Lord. Shouldn't Jesus and I be sitting on a Victorian, cast iron bench in a lush garden—you know that hymn, "*I come to the garden alone where the dew is still on the roses... And He walks with me and He talks with me and He tells me I am His own. And the joy we share as we tarry there, none other has ever known.*" What about that?

G: I create opportunities for those beautiful experiences, too. However, I am asking you to conceive of something different. Just you and Jesus on that grey bench with nothing else and no one else to see, feel, hear, taste, or touch. Can you still hear his voice telling you, "*I am with you. You can do this?*"

L: I am trying.

G: Lisa, I have noticed how you like to read John's description of Jesus in the book of Revelation. Remember how he describes Jesus' voice as the *sound of rushing waters* (Rev. 1:15, NIV)?

Imagine the most glorious waterfall you have ever experienced. Remember how the sound of ocean waves satisfies you at your very core? Now imagine hearing Jesus say with a voice of those glorious waters, *"I am with you, Lisa. You can do this."*

L: Whoa. I am beginning to understand. I think this is where the Psalmist would write *"Selah"*—I will pause, abide, and receive.

I invite you to pause with me a moment and imagine Jesus' voice as rushing waters. What other descriptions of Jesus from the Bible could you more fully integrate into your life?

Simply Jesus: Okay With Grey

L: I feel helpless, weak, overwhelmed. I want to give up. I can't keep going. What do you want me to remember and appreciate, Lord?

G: How about you and Jesus on the bench?

L: Ahhh, that secret and slightly uncomfortable place. You know how much I want more of Jesus. I want this to be my favorite place, but you know how much I dislike grey. I need the yellow of sunshine, the blues and teals of the water, the greens of the grass and trees. You made such incredible colors. I know they do something great for my brain, my soul, my spirit.

G: Thank you. Yes, I am glad you enjoy the colors. I love watching you sigh and breathe deep when you are on the water, always appreciating my blues and greens. I know how much joy you have felt these past two decades bringing your daughters to recreate in nature—the ocean, to Acadia National Park, to your parent's home and on favorite hikes? I feel that same joy when you revel in my colors and nature. I hope you keep enjoying them. However, I invite you to consider this. What if you could simply enjoy Jesus?

L: I thought I did. You have more for me, don't you?

G: Of course! Every time you tell me you are longing for more of Jesus, I set you up to receive more.

L: Good to know. Thank you for paying attention to my desires and preparing me to receive them. I love singing that Chris Tomlin song to you: *"All of you is more than enough for all of me. For every thirst and every need, You satisfy me with Your love, and all I have in You is more than enough."*[1]

G: And I love hearing you sing it to me. Remember what else is in John's description of Jesus in chapter one of Revelation: *"His eyes were like blazing fire."* What if your body felt as warm and comforted by Jesus looking into your eyes as you do when you stare at red and yellow flames in a fireplace dancing across your line of vision?

I notice how much you are drawn to the sun. You open every curtain; you move around to sit by a window. You do anything you can to feel the sun shining on your face and in your eyes. When Jesus sits next to you on the grey bench, puts His arm around you, and tells you, *"I am with you, Lisa. You can do this."* His face is *"like the sun shining in all its brilliance"* (Rev. 1:16, NIV). What would it be like for you to soak up His presence, His encouragement, His validation, and His inspiration the same way you soak up the sun?

L: Hmm, I like thinking this way and experiencing you like this, Jesus. My resilience is kicking in, and I feel more capable, strengthened, and confident. It is as if I am throwing a heavy

---

1. Tomlin, Chris. *"Enough."* YouTube. https://www.youtube.com/watch?v=87Ig-lnWjzQ.

rug off my back, getting up from the floor and walking forward again. I am beginning to be ok with grey. You are in the grey.

You Can't Afford Not to Do This

L: Here I am again, back on this bench with Jesus. This time I am surrounded by comrades from my leader team. We are taking turns sharing stories as we interact in our secret places with you. I am juggling emotions on opposite sides of the spectrum. I feel anxious, timid, and overwhelmed with decisions. This restless energy in my body needs a channel to run through and a productive outcome. At the same time, I feel hopeful. The memory bank in my brain contains ample evidence that when I am with these people who also desire to connect with you, we all feel happier and wiser by the end of our gathering.

G: Isn't it great how I can be fully present and attentive to each one of you at the same time?

L: Yes. It is so rejuvenating to get closer to you even as I hear how others are doing that simultaneously. It seems as though we are all seeing more of you more clearly. I am living out the answer to Paul's prayer to the Ephesians: *"And I pray that you, being rooted and established in love, may have power, together with all the Lord's holy people, to grasp how wide and long and high and deep is the love of Christ, and to know this love that surpasses knowledge- that you may be filled to the measure of all the fullness of God" (Ephesians 3:17-19, NIV).*

G: What are you hearing from Jesus now as He sits right next to you and coaches you?

L: Jesus is telling me, *"You can do this, Lisa. You cannot afford not to do this. You can stand up from this bench and bring your best true self to the world around you."* I know this is true. I cannot afford not to move forward. I won't shrink back or give up. The cost is too great.

Later that day...

Honor Instead of Shame

L: I am still thinking about our leadership training gathering today and how satisfied and refreshed I feel.

G: Did you notice that when you shared these words with the rest of the group how impacted they were? You don't know all the details and outcomes in their lives, but by simply being with me and sharing what you are hearing and experiencing with me, you are giving others courage to stand up, take risks, and be their best, true selves.

L: This is how I want to be a leader and an elder. I didn't give any advice. We didn't even get all tangled up in the messy details of each other's lives and the obstacles we are navigating. We just came straight to you, interacting honestly and authentically, sharing the most important parts about our interactions with you. We gave each other space to take in what we heard from you and each other and applied it as we needed it. This is so honoring.

G: I love how you are valuing your heart's desire for honor. This is who I created you to be. You honor me when you live out the values I put inside you. Honor is propagated and noticed. It's an honor party!

L: You know how often I have begged you to answer the promise of Isaiah 61:7 that Jesus came to fulfill: *"Instead of shame and dishonor, you will enjoy a double share of honor"* for all the people and situations I hold close to my heart, including myself. I didn't realize it would look like this. It is becoming so natural as it flows out of my relationship with you and others.

G: Here is the *"easy button,"* brought to you by Jesus!

What a joy to be simultaneously experiencing growth as a participant in a leader team, the facilitator of leader teams, and as an individual who continually is being surprised, strengthened, and taught by God. This next series of interactions changed my life. How grateful I am that I took time to listen in the presence of a listening coach just for the adventure of learning, even though I wasn't in a crisis or desperately needing help.

From the Sailboat to the Mirror

L: What do you want me to remember today, God?

G: When you were six years old, your parents' big sailboat was on the lawn in the backyard. Your dad picked you up and sat you on the bow. You were coloring in a coloring book when your mom took a picture of you.

L: Yes, I remember that. I used to love looking at that picture. I liked the way my light brown hair sloped down smoothly, partially covering my cheek and curling at the ends. It looked so sophisticated. I loved how I was thinking outside the box by using a sailboat bow as my craft table. The white sail was hoisted, shading me from the sun and serving as my backdrop. Behind the sailboat was a pastoral view of green trees, the valley below, and blue skies dotted with fluffy clouds. My legs were gracefully extended and crossed at the ankles, with my feet pointed slightly in my stylish brown sandals, foreshadowing that they belonged to a future ballerina.

I have many happy memories sailing in that sailboat, so I found great pleasure in sitting on it off-season. Every time I looked at that photo something deep in me said, *"This is me. This is who I've always been. Look at me being me."* I feel happy, strong, and confident now, and I remember feeling that way every time I looked at that picture.

G: I also took pleasure seeing you coloring on the sailboat with the support of your mom and dad. I was with you every time you pulled that photo out.

L: You and I seem to be transcending time and space.

G: Yes. That is what I am like, and when you look at life through my eyes, you understand that more deeply. I look at you and that photo and say, *"I know. I know. This is who you are and who you always will be. Those things that you like about yourself—I like them, too."*

L: I can tell you are delighting in me. I can see it in your face. I feel warm and bright like the sun is shining on my insides. [Chuckling] It's like that phrase, *"I've got sunshine in my pocket"* from the song, *"Can't Stop the Feeling."* What do you want me to know about this? Why am I remembering this today?

G: I want you to remember that you can always be young at heart like you were on the sailboat. You don't even have to look at that photo to have that light shining inside. You can look at me now and have it any time and all the time.

L: Ooh, that touches a tender spot, which was deeply buried in me. I didn't even realize what was going on inside me until now. It feels so important that you noticed me on the sailboat and that you were in tune with me, liking what I liked about myself through the years as I looked at this photo.

G: Yes, what is going on in your heart, Lisa?

L: I feel so vulnerable as I get older. It is so hard not to have my body work like it used to. I have always relied on my body and my ability to be strong, flexible, and always moving. With my kinesthetic learning style, I learn, think, and get inspired best while I am moving, walking, dancing, running, doing chores, swimming, or biking. You have miraculously healed my body six times. Now I feel aches and pains and legitimate reasons to be cautious and inhibited. Getting old is scary and full of vulnerability. It will only get harder. Although I don't obsess about my looks, I realize now that I certainly don't look at myself with the same pleasure as I once did. How I wish I could look at myself and feel the same way I did when admiring that six-year-old.

Now as I think of my mom and others whom I care about who struggle with chronic pain, fatigue, injury, and illness, I understand how susceptible they feel as their strength and energy declines. I feel tender and sad. Is there anything else you want me to know about that?

G: I know what it is like to feel vulnerable in my body. I became a human baby. I endured torture and crucifixion. I experienced losing strength and power even though I didn't experience getting old. I needed to completely rely on others when I left my Father's side and entered earth as a baby. During my crucifixion, I was utterly exposed and defenseless.

L: I feel speechless and in awe of you, Jesus.

G: Please absorb the reality that I also proceeded to defeat death and live forever. Your new reality is that I will stay with you, walk with you, and see you through the rest of your life. I can't take away your sadness or the natural effects of aging, but I can be with you, give you access to a new strength, and ease your sadness.

L: This feels scary and reassuring at the same time.

G: I am always here with you, looking at you and delighting in you no matter what age and no matter what stage of life. Let's shift from the sailboat on the lawn to your bathroom.

L: My bathroom?

G: Do you know that when you stand in the bathroom and glance in the mirror every day, I am right behind you looking over your right shoulder and seeing you in the mirror? I feel the same delight now that I felt each time we looked at the photo of you coloring on the sailboat.

L: Wow! You are with me in my bathroom mirror? Heck, I am barely with me in my bathroom mirror. This feels so real and true and yet such a new thought to remember that you are with me even in my bathroom mirror. I will take this to heart.

This was truly life-altering. Now I am unable to mindlessly rush through my morning routine. Although I have never invested much time or money in skin care products, I am enticed by Jesus to STOP and feel the lotion on my face and to tenderly touch my face while absorbing Jesus' love into my body. When I attempt my multi-tasking swirl of brushing teeth, putting clothes in the laundry basket, looking for matching socks, I am compelled to STOP.

I return to the mirror and have this quiet, solidifying moment with God. It is as if God is authorizing me to be myself, as I sense His complete attention, compassion, and delight toward me. I concur with Him by choosing these little nurturing acts of self-care and self-awareness. I feel endorsed and authenticated as if God and I both signed a permission slip for me to be myself in the world that day. I can better grasp what Paul meant when he wrote to the Corinthians:

"That is why we never give up. Though our bodies are dying, our spirits are being renewed every day. For our present troubles are small and won't last long. Yet they produce for us a glory that vastly outweighs them and will last forever" (2 Corinthians 4: 16, NLT).

More on the Mirror

G: How are you feeling as you look in the mirror and see Me seeing you?

L: Amazed, validated, relaxed, and peaceful.

G: Good. Now, is there any part of you rejecting this idea?

L: Yes, the twenty-year-old me who wanted to accomplish so many things and make such an impact on the world and who was so gifted, capable, and adventurous—that part of me feels sad, like my best years have passed.

G: Hmm. I am with you in your sadness. Do you really believe your best years have passed?

L: It is hard to say. I change my mind with every change of circumstance.

G: Is there anything else you are feeling?

L: Yes, actually, I feel ANGRY! I feel ripped off. I fell for a lie. Somewhere along the way, I accepted the message: "*You can hit the fountain of youth with Jesus.*" I feel angry at those who taught this and put on a show about it. I feel angry at myself for believing it. What do I need to know about this anger? What do you want me to do with it?

G: I invented anger. There's no need to be afraid of it, and I don't want you to stuff it. I invite you to convert your anger into fuel. Use it as energy toward change. I have a better way to grow old. You can use that fuel to position yourself to receive my grace and trust me with every upcoming day of your life.

L: You don't give us the fountain of youth on this side of heaven, but you give us the capacity to grow old without losing heart. I am thinking about that same verse as before in a different version: *"Therefore we do not lose heart. Though outwardly we are wasting away, yet inwardly we are being renewed day by day"* (2 Corinthians 4:16, NIV).

L: I want that, please!

Earning my health coach certification demanded that I become more compassionate toward my weaknesses and more audacious in my self-care. Small yet indispensable steps of caring for my body became the gateway for caring for my soul and stepping into more of God's love.

Just Drink Water

L: Oh, it is time to get up, and I am full of dread. I hardly slept. How can I face this day? I feel full of grief and shame about how my fear and fatigue impacted our rare and special family time this weekend. Now I will have to say goodbye to them within the next few hours. Time has run out for restoring things to the way I hoped they would be. There is no time for me to even be still with you, yet I need our time together to move forward and not fail further. What can I do? How can I take care of myself right now in these few moments so I can handle this day and love my family?

G: Drink your water. You take care of yourself by drinking your water first thing every morning, and you coach your clients to do the same.

L: Yes, it is such an easy and effective way to start the day.

G: Let me love and restore you through the water you will drink now.

L: Okay. Thanks for making it that easy.

G: From now on, this simple act of drinking water can be another way of nourishing your soul and being with me.

L: Just like being with you in the bathroom mirror.

G: You really are catching on about making our relationship easy, simple, and part of everyday life.

L: I always love to maximize the benefits of every opportunity. Now drinking water, brushing my teeth, and washing my face have become special times with you that empower me and give my life value. This reminds me of when Paul invited the Ephesians to: *"Be careful then how you live, not as unwise people but as wise, making the most of the time, because the days are evil."* (Ephesians 5:15,16, NRSV).

G: Yes, and remember that you can be both careful and carefree with me.

~~~

Juggling the seemingly opposite characteristics of careful and carefree enticed me, especially as I sought to emerge from confused to confident.
~~~

CHAPTER 4

I Can See Clearly Now

From Confused to Confident

Resilience—The ability to spring back into shape after being compressed[1]

My daughters tease me that I have a song for everything. I love to break out and sing a few key lines of a song to reinforce what we are thinking, feeling, or wondering about. I love God's sense of humor and how much He validates my life by playing my song. Often when I ask Him, *"What do you want me to know?"* lyrics from a song pop into my head. Frankly, I pay just as much attention to the *"non-spiritual"* songs that require me to think deeply

1. Dictionary.com, compiled from two definitions.

about which words are meant for me and why. Plus, I get a lot of joy out of playing an old tune, singing loudly, and dancing freely. Sometimes, that truly feels like church because my perspective shifts, and I see God more clearly. So I asked God:

L: Why are you reminding me of all these random old songs from the past that are not even overtly Christian songs?

G: I know how much you and your family love singing to me and dancing to songs about me, and I know how excruciating it is for you to be triggered with painful memories and paralyzed from singing.

L: Thank you for noticing. I miss singing with other people so much, but it can become so confusing and painful that my anxiety increases, and I feel further disconnected from you and others. What a mess!

G: I am reminding you of these songs so you would find another way to sing to me and with me. I want to find a way for you to keep singing because I created you to enjoy that.

L: Wow. Thank you so much. You are so good, so resourceful, so creative, and so open-minded.

G: I love you, and I want the best for you. I want you to know that I see every part of your life, and I know all the songs from every era for all time.

L: You are amazing.

~~~

I was fifty-one years old and desperate for clarity after a really confusing time and a profound identity crisis. The song that came in my head was from the '70s— "I Can See Clearly Now." It seemed like God was nudging me to trust Him and myself and believe that
~~~

I could make sense of life, discern what was true from what was counterfeit, and dance on my own two feet like a little girl standing on her daddy's feet, waltzing with Him.

I made an empowering discovery during a two-day coaching intensive on accessing my true design; I can trust my instincts.[2] *In order to acknowledge and value that intuition is a legitimate tool I possess when coaching others, I needed to first re-establish my identity, listen to my own voice, and value my perceptivity. Prior to that, some internal housecleaning of my theology was also necessary. Following are some of the conversations that cleared the smog off my spiritual eyes.*

~~~

Seeing Me as Me

While attending a conference to inaugurate the season of Lent, I identified and removed a big obstacle, which was hindering my ability to grow deeper and closer to God. Much applause goes to the conference speakers and planners who allowed two hours after lunch to reflect with God and integrate the lectures we heard that morning.[3] *The following conversation occurred in this two-hour window.*

L: The last talk I heard explained that some teach and preach the message that you don't actually love us. You really only love Jesus in us. My left brain seems to say that I never in all my years of studying scripture, listening to sermons, and training at seminary heard such an unsound and erroneous message,

2. Coach Tim Morris, https://designdiscovery.com/
3. Betsy Stalcup, https://www.godhealstoday.org/ and David Tackle, https://kingdomformation.org/
~~~

but my right brain is alerting me to pay attention and dislodge something deep in my heart.

G: I am here with you, patiently waiting to hear what you discover in your heart. You can come to me with anything and everything.

L: I feel so tender and cautious being with you now. It is as if I am on this plank walking toward you. I want to get to you without falling off, so I need to step carefully. This is a very tenuous place.

G: I love you, and I see you, Lisa. I love you for who you are. I care for you specifically and intentionally. I like to look at you and see you being you and doing what gives you joy because I made you that way. I am delighted when you are fully alive.

L: That makes sense to me. What doesn't make sense is this notion that when you look at me you only see Jesus and that you merely tolerate me because of Jesus.

G: That is not meant to make sense.

L: Ugh! It feels as though I am in the middle of childbirth—the pains of delivery. It is as if I am struggling to birth a new life. What is going on?

G: I am here with you. Take your time to figure it out. It will be worth it.

L: If I believe this somehow, then it logically follows that I must also believe that Jesus is keeping me from you. It is as if Jesus is an obstacle between us instead of the One who makes it possible for all of us to know each other.

G: What do you think and how do you feel about that?

L: I feel confused. I must somehow have this hidden resentment of you, Jesus, for getting between God and me. How awful,

Jesus, I am sorry—so, so sorry. You are not blocking me from God. You have cleared the way for me to be intimate with you, God my Daddy, and Holy Spirit. Thank you for what you have done for me. How could I ever have buried this resentment toward you? Please forgive me for harboring this resentment. I feel so bewildered and sad.

G: I forgive you, Lisa. This barrier is no longer between us.

L: Wow. It feels like the pain has passed. The delivery is over. I have given birth to this new life with you. I feel peace and calm in my core. The tension in my gut has dissolved.

G: I feel sad that you have been stuck in this confusion, and I feel angry that others representing me have taught this.

L: Thank you for connecting with me and helping me understand your feelings, too.

G: I have always been with you. I love you. I see you. I want you to know that anything that you didn't receive because you were wrestling with this conflict deep down will all be restored to you. You and I will experience intimacy with nothing holding you back, and it will be as if nothing ever held you back as you continue to walk with me and enjoy being with me.

L: I believe you. I feel seen. I remember the painting of Jesus I stared at just minutes ago.[4]

G: I see you letting yourself be seen by me. Would you let me continue to remind you of how I have been with you your whole life?

L: Yes, I want that.

4. Painting by Akiane Kramarik: https://art-soulworks.com/collections/prince-of-peace

G: Would you let me show you how I see you now and how I see your life?

L: Yes, I want that. I feel restored, but tired. I am going to lie on a church pew and rest with you with nothing between us. My left and right brain, my heart, my soul, and my body, all of them tell me, "*This is good and right. I am being me. You are being you. We are seeing each other as we truly are.*"

G: Rest well, daughter.

I did indeed rest well. Although my husband and I were at odds, he found me on the pew, obtained a blanket and laid it over me. I gladly received his kindness and the gift of being seen by a human. I emerged with my heart and mind engaged to wrestle more and receive every truth and blessing I could from God. A mentor once pointed out that "rest" is in the middle of "wrestle": wRESTle. My conversation continued:

He Sees Me Hidden with Christ in God

L: I still want to learn everything I need to about that false idea. I wonder if there are other Bible verses that I distorted to back-up that notion.

G: Great question. Is anything coming to mind?

L: Well, I often used to think about that verse, which says, "*For you died and your life is now hidden with Christ in God*" (Colossians 3:3, NIV). I wonder if somehow I applied it in a way that is similar to erasing myself.

G: Well, let's make sure you see yourself as bold, vibrant, and noticeable. What do you think that verse really means?

L: Thanks for asking. I think it means that my life is wrapped up in you. I am surrounded by you. I am no longer like a flailing, unswaddled baby. I never can go beyond your reach and care.

G: I like it. What do you think has died?

L: What has died:

The part of me that thinks I can live only with my own power.

The part of me that thinks I can save myself.

The part of me that is hopelessly and frantically trying to make sense of life.

The part of me that wants to be someone else or something different, something less than or something more than who you created me to be.

The part of me that thinks I can make sense of the world, that I could judge good and evil and others' motives or that I could see anything clearly apart from you.

When I let all that die and keep myself hidden in you because of Jesus, then I feel warm and fully alive. I am seen. I am willing and able to make sense of life from your perspective.

G: Yes, yes, yes. I see you, love you, and agree with you.

Where Did That Come From?

L: Jesus, I know that you are not an obstacle blocking me from God. You are not in the way. You are the way.

G: Yes, [smiling] *"the way, the truth, and the life"* (John 14:6, NIV).

L: I don't remember where I heard that teaching about God looking at me and only loving Jesus in me, not me. Where did I get that idea? Where did I hear that?

About six weeks after the conference, at the end of a delightful and inspiring Easter service, the pastor said in his final benediction, "Remember when God looks at you, He sees Jesus."

L: Ahhh, found it! That is where that came from. How disappointing that this happened after such a wonderful service. Thank you, God, that I am no longer bound by this message. Thank you that your love and truth prevents me from absorbing an ounce of it. Thank you that you look at me and see me because of Jesus. Thank you that there is *"no veil between us"* (Solomon's Song of Songs 1:7, TPT). Please restore truth to all the others who internalized this message, and show me if there is something I can do about that.

After experiencing pain, followed by restoration and clarity with God, I felt more drawn to and hopeful about interacting with Him about other obstacles that kept me from seeing Him clearly. It became easier and easier to go to Him with my questions and feelings.

Untangling the Nest

L: Even though we solved that issue about you seeing me, my brain is still out of sorts.

G: There will always be more to sort out on this side of Heaven. I am with you, and I am happy to talk about more issues. What is out of sorts?

L: It is as if my brain is like a nest. Nests are supposed to be comprised of simple, organic materials that birds pick up in nature. Yet the nest I see has all this junk in it. There's trash, debris, plastic bottle caps, straws, and cigarette butts. It is all tangled up in the nest. God, please show me what you are doing with my brain?

G: I am coming like a mother bird and pulling out the junk in the nest. I am unraveling the plastic twine that is wrapped around debris and recreating the nest to be a place of rest and protection and growth.

L: I feel peaceful and hopeful imagining that you could do this for me. I want my mind to be a place where others can be with me, feel at home, and settle into a resting place. I want my mind to be a place of hospitality for myself and for others.

G: We will work on it together, you and I. I know you have the heart of a mother bird. Your nest will be restored and many baby birds will rest, grow, eat, and fly from the welcoming environment of growth that you will offer.

L: Let it be so, God. I feel comforted and hopeful envisioning this

One of the most significant ways my "nest" was cleaned out occurred during a long drive in the middle of my transition to empty nest.

Prayer Decluttering via Matthew 6

After dropping my youngest daughter off for the summer in Ohio, knowing she would only return for one week at the end of summer before moving out, I faced a six-hour drive home and felt oddly ambivalent about returning to Virginia. My husband and other daughter (who only visited for a few nights at a time while on college break) were leaving the next day for a two-week trip to Asia with his side of the family. It felt as though returning home was like dropping into a black hole. I knew my only hope was experiencing Jesus in a more tangible way. The most sensible strategy, while driving in the car, was to listen to stories of Jesus' life when he walked this earth. I listened to the audio version of Matthew from "The Message" over and over for several hours. Rather than being bored, I was undone.

As I listened to chapter six in the book of Matthew, I was overcome by grief, yet compelled to listen. There was a massive decluttering going on in my mind as Jesus identified with painful precision many ideas and practices on how to pray that I had diligently accumulated over the years. Following is just one of the conversations we had on that cleansing drive:

"The world is full of so-called prayer warriors who are prayer-ignorant. They're full of formulas and programs and advice, peddling techniques for getting what you want from God. Don't fall for that nonsense. This is your Father you are dealing with, and he knows better than you what you need" (Matthew 6:7, MSG).

L: I did fall for that. I feel so sorry, so sad, and so regretful. I can think of so many times when my children were in pain. I felt so vulnerable and needy, and I just wanted to find a quick solution. Oh, all those books, courses, workshops, conferences, methods, and prayers I invested in—convinced that I had finally found our solution. All the time I spent learning what things to say and not say when praying.

Ugh, it all feels so complicated. I am sorry for all the ways I became reliant on that instead of you. I am sorry for all the ways I easily blamed something or someone else and called it prayer. I am sorry I didn't learn how to genuinely endure pain and how to simply be with others in their pain. I am sorry for how I cut myself off from my own heart and certainly from yours. I am sorry for the times I modeled to my children that prayer is complicated.

G: I forgive you. I know how painful this is for you, how big this is, and how sorry you are. We will figure it out together. Your family saw your true heart and you did model that you love me and rely on me. You already apologized to them for when you made prayer complicated, and they forgave you. I can relieve you of these burdens whenever you say the word.

L: Yes, please relieve me of these burdens of guilt and shame. Thank you for forgiving me. I feel forgiven. Thank you for leading me out and drawing me to you. Thank you that there is nothing between us, that I can just simply be with you. I feel completely emptied. Please help me learn to pray all over again.

G: *"With a God like (me) loving you, you can pray very simply. Like this: Our Father in heaven, Reveal who you are. Set the world right; Do what's best—as above, so below. Keep us alive with three square meals. Keep us forgiven with you and forgiving others. Keep us safe from ourselves and the Devil. You're in charge! You can do anything you want! You're ablaze in beauty! Yes. Yes. Yes"* (Matthew 6:9-13, MSG).

L: You are taking me by the hand and leading me out with this prayer. Since you said to pray like this, I will use each of these points to help me access my heart and my mind as I converse with you. I want you to be my teacher and trainer. Yes, please teach me to pray, Jesus.

This experience inaugurated a season where I pictured Jesus as my Good Shepherd, holding my hand as we walked along green pastures as He said one phrase of this prayer at a time. I took long, deep breaths between each line and then interacted with God based on that line.

For example, I just took a writing break and followed my Good Shepherd's lead in using His prayer as my guide. I like to pause and take slow, deep breaths after each new thought:

L: "*Our Father in heaven, hallowed be your name*—Help me, God. I have so much to learn about how holy you are and how there is no one like you. Help me continually learn more about who you truly are and to love you uniquely in a way that honors you as you.

Your kingdom come, your will be done, on earth as it is in heaven—Your kingdom is described as one of "*righteousness, peace and joy*" (Romans 14:7, NRSV). Could you please surround and inspire my daughters with righteousness, peace and joy through people and organizations?

Give us today our daily bread—Help me realize what I need and ask you for it. *extra breath* I feel this strong need to justify myself in a certain situation. Please help me set it aside until more information and clarity is revealed.

And forgive us our debts—I feel resentment toward _____. Please forgive me.

As we also have forgiven our debtors—I forgive that same person for their actions toward me.

And lead us not into temptation—I feel tempted to hide and refrain from speaking up about a concern. Please help me see more clearly from your perspective, and then give me courage to speak.

But deliver us from the evil one—You know this situation that seems so evil and troubling to me. Please fight that battle in the way that only you can.

I continued to use the Lord's Prayer as a tool, like a walking stick, on my journey with Jesus. Fortunately, before we became empty nesters, our family adopted this prayer into our evening routine complete with the long, deep breaths. When it stayed within the boundaries of being a conversation starter with God, it helped me persevere with the open, spontaneous conversations that we have.

You Can Do This!

L: God, I feel so many conflicting feelings today that I am overwhelmed, paralyzed, and stuck. What do you want me to remember?

G: On the first day of summer girl scout camp, when you were eight years old, the bus driver stopped at the end of a road and impatiently told you to get off.

L: Yes, I was shocked and unable to speak up and tell her it was a really long walk in the hot sun to get to my house and this must be a mistake. I got off the bus and started walking on a rural road with few houses. I planned to get myself to the house of a family friend and ask for help if they were home. As they were driving home, they noticed me. I got into the car and collapsed in the arms of my friend's grandma, even though I didn't know her well. She held me as I cried. My fear and sadness shifted to comfort and relief, and I felt rescued, reassured, and peaceful. I knew I would be okay, and it would not happen again. They cooled me off with a popsicle and cold water, called my mom, and she picked me up.

G: I had my arms around you and the grandma holding you. I saw what happened and made sure someone would come for you.

L: I feel some shame now. Why didn't I speak up and tell the bus driver I was too far from home to walk? Why did I let her anger and impatience intimidate me?

G: I know that was a hard time for you, and I am glad you remembered how you returned to joy and peace from fear and sadness. You did a good job making a plan, even though you didn't speak up. I am not ashamed of you for not speaking up, Lisa. That would have been a lot to ask of an eight-year-old, and you didn't have that skill developed yet.

L: Thank you. I feel peaceful knowing you are not ashamed of me. I have certainly had plenty of opportunities to learn to speak up even when I felt intimidated. Yet, I would like to grow even more.

G: You can practice on me.

L: Okay. I want to talk about this memory that I have thought about over and over. It is like bad bowling. The neural pathways in my brain seem to have formed a side track that the gutter ball stays in. I have tried over and over to reframe this. I have sought help from others, taken countless courses on healing, and learned so many strategies. Can we try again?

G: Of course, I love your tenacity. I love that you come to me and believe we can find the solution together. You are completely free to speak up.

L: Please help me. I am eager to see my life from your perspective.

G: What part of your life are you looking at?

L: The first month when I was a preemie in an incubator in the hospital.

G: What would you like to see?

L: I have learned so much about how crucial it is for a newborn baby to immediately bond with a mother or caregiver. Since this could not happen from an incubator, I have worried so much about my deficiencies. Additionally, I have replayed and magnified the stories in my mind about how difficult this was for my parents. I have wrestled with the confusion of how I could be both too much and not enough. I have heard others tell stories of seeing you looking at them while they were in the incubator. Why can't I see that? Why can't you show me your face?

G: Do you want to adopt their story or do you want to know yours?

L: Argh. Okay, I want to know my story.

G: Can you see where I am and sense what I am doing and saying?

L: NO. All I sense is the frenzy. This doesn't make any sense. I see Jesus trying to race around with my mom on the forty-five-minute drive to the hospital, exhausted and stressed. She is overwhelmed with the pressure to get me to eat enough so I can gain weight and go home. I sense Jesus hurrying with my dad to manage his business, finish the nursery since I arrived early, and see me in the hospital. Now I am picking up the frenzy. This does not make sense.

G: How are you feeling?

L: I feel vulnerable, anxious, and full of hopeless despair. I see myself as this flailing, unswaddled baby. I can't soothe myself or swaddle myself. Where are you? What do I need to know?

G: Lisa, somehow I got you from that incubator in the hospital to where you are today. I brought you from there to here. What would it take for you to know that I had you then, I rescued you eight years later when your friends picked you up and held you as you cried, and I have you now? Not only that, I will have you in the future.

L: That feels like a huge paradigm shift. There's a whole lot of blank space in my mind where I don't know what happened. Can I really just concentrate on the places where I can see you and not all the places I can't?

I need a Selah pause to reflect on that. Would you join me?

I would love to have seen a scan of my brain from this encounter because I imagine it was like plugging in a string of lights at Christmas as new neural pathways were created. Recognizing and enlarging God's presence started becoming a habit that I chose because I knew the benefits far exceeded the cost. I began to ask God to show me any memory He wanted to without a lot of filters and requirements because I trusted Him more. I felt confident that He wanted to remind me of something so I could remember that He was with me.

There Must Be Something There That Wasn't There Before

L: So I have been singing that song from *Beauty and the Beast*, "*There Must Be Something There That Wasn't There Before.*" I am getting used to the idea that you were the *something* there. You were always there, although I didn't perceive it.

G: I am glad you paid attention to me when I sang that song for you.

L: So is there anything you want me to know about when I was a premature baby in the incubator at the hospital? I am sorry for demanding to see your face.

G: No worries, Lisa. I forgive you.

L: I want to see what you have for me to see. What was there that I couldn't see before?

G: First, consider this. How would you as an adult respond to that little premature baby?

L: The baby? I would pick her up and hold her just like I did with my two daughters. I would feel so much joy, and I would smile at her and show her how completely and utterly thrilled I was to be holding her and seeing her.

As soon as I imagined picking myself up as a baby. I could sense Jesus with me in a very specific way.

L: Ahhh—I see Jesus now. You are kneeling on the hospital floor with your hands on my knees. You are admiring me, the baby, and your face is beaming at me, the momma. The fire of courage and pride is burning in your eyes as you smile at me, the momma. My soul is warmed to the core.

G: You can do this, Lisa! You can do this! I am so proud of you. Look what you did. You took the baby, wrapped the baby up, and loved her. You did just what I would do because you have my heart! This is your story. First, you needed to see yourself as an adult caring for yourself as a baby, then you were able to see me.

L: It is like you are integrating me through all the stages of my life. I feel surprisingly different, alive, and validated—ready to face the world. I feel strong enough to dismiss the accusations that I am not a good mom. The little, premature baby in me feels soothed, quieted, and comforted even if there is frenzy around me. The younger mother in me feels affirmed, empowered, noticed, and coached by Jesus.

G: I feel so happy for you. Can you see the difference this reframe will make in your life?

L: Yes, whenever I feel stuck or ashamed, I can stop and remember this reality. I can make my decisions and move forward with them. I can hear myself saying, "*We can do this!*" and see you nodding enthusiastically. My body feels strong and reliable.

G: Let's keep moving forward!

During a missions trip to Brazil four years ago, I dreamt that I was walking through an old cabin. A long, rustic table was lined with dusty mason jars filled with rocks. I had the sense that I was being invited to open the jars and find the beauty and hidden treasures nestled in between the rocks. I was beginning to mine out the hidden treasures and started asking God to show me beauty.

I See the Race You Are Running

L: Could you please show me something beautiful?

G: Remember when you were in your mid-twenties and house sitting on Cousins Island? You would run from Cousins Island to Little John Island.

L: Yes, I remember one fall day when the sun was shining and the air was warm enough for shorts and a T-shirt but cool enough to be brisk and energizing. You know how much I love feeling the sun on my face! My body felt strong and free as I ran with nothing holding me back. My gaze shifted between the ocean view with the sparkling water multiplying the light, the lobster boats puttering around, and the gliding sailboats. On land, I noticed the split rail fences, the swooshes of black-eyed Susans, and puffs of orange, purple, and burgundy mums.

For the first time in my life, I distinctly knew that you were noticing me, even when I wasn't trying to get anyone's attention.

G: Yes, I told you, "Lisa I see you. I watched you all those years that you ran your cross-country and track races, when you ran for the team, the crowd, your coach, and your family. I noticed how hard you worked, how disciplined and dedicated you were, and how you pushed your body to the limit. Today, I see you even though no one else is looking. I see your ponytail dancing and circling, your lavender shorts and white T-shirt.

L: I didn't even realize I needed to be seen, but I feel so much more alive and energized knowing you saw me that day.

G: Why do you think I am reminding you of this today?

L: Please, tell me why.

G: Lisa, I am still noticing the race you are running. I am proud of you. Keep going. You are running well.

L: Wow. I wasn't expecting this. I feel stronger and more confident to face the hard things of life—much harder than finishing a cross-country race. Thank you for seeing me and connecting these dots of real moments in my life.

G: I am all about connecting the dots!

~~~

The prerequisite to recognizing and appreciating beauty requires a heart that can feel. The next chapter will reveal the work I did in overcoming obstacles and giving myself permission to feel.
~~~

CHAPTER 5

Can't Stop the Feeling

Ambivalent to Alive

"Lord, who fully knows the power of your passion and the intensity of your emotions?" —Psalm 90:11, TPT

Several years ago, my husband and I embarked on a week-long intensive, evaluating our lives from several angles and identifying obstacles that were hindering our growth and maturity. As a result, we determined that we would no longer suppress our negative emotions or dismiss them in each other. On our first night home, we instituted a new routine of asking specific questions about how we were feeling at dinner, and our daughters responded with, *"This is so awkward!"*

It was a clumsy time as we all tried to learn to live from our hearts more authentically and accept the bad and the ugly more graciously. The timing was amazing because after that first dinner, my daughters picked out the children's movie *Frozen* for us to watch. Elsa, the main character was afflicted with a destructive, magical power that froze everything she touched. Her anger and fear of hurting those she loved escalated when loss, hardship, and situations beyond her control overwhelmed her. She ran away, created her own ice tower, and became a recluse singing, *"The cold doesn't bother me anyway."* On the brink of death, Elsa's survival required her to receive her younger sister's love and risk the pain involved in being close to her, knowing she might hurt her. I joked with my daughters for choosing the perfect movie to go with our new efforts to be more real with our feelings.

A few years later, our family heartily embraced and enjoyed the movie *Inside Out* and realized how much we had grown up out of our awkward stage. The movie producers and script writers brilliantly distilled some of the discoveries in brain science and validated the way we were navigating all our emotions, especially sadness.

It has certainly been challenging to be on the accelerated track of not only accepting emotions, but also expressing and managing them.

By then, I had acquired just enough tools to start dealing with a barrage of events that warranted much grief and sadness. The grief I accessed deep in my gut was best expressed through wails and tears. This created a second problem; the anxious anticipation that I might break out with those wails and tears in the grocery store. Since I couldn't blame this on menopause (been there, done that), I resolved to dig deeper. I sought to learn everything I could about myself and talk with God about how to cope. When I asked God:

L: What do I need in order to be my true self without shame? How do I live from my heart, feel deeply, and grieve authentically without giving up, shutting back down, and getting depressed?

I sensed Him saying two things:

G: Forbearance and self-regulation.

Following are conversations with God about the major emotions identified as fear, anger, disgust, shame, hopeless despair, and sadness. I appreciate how Bill St. Cyr of Ambleside Schools refers to them as protector emotions rather than negative emotions.[1] This validates that our Creator gave us these emotions for a purpose. When we let them alert us to pay attention and respond appropriately, we take care of ourselves and each other and honor our Creator. These conversations reveal how, once I could see my situation from God's perspective, I was then able to regulate the intensity of the emotions. As I turned the intensity down a notch, I was also able to turn up the dial on my peace and joy. God and I collaborated on pulling me out of the ditch so I could get back on track and stay connected with Him and others.

This first conversation occurred six years ago. I remember it whenever I feel tempted to make a U-turn and numb out from this adventurous road trip. God is talking less in this conversation because I was still learning to recognize how He was with me consistently. This is a great example of how He gave me the perseverance to continue looking and listening for Him without giving up.

1. https://www.amblesideschools.com/blog/teacher-homeschool/specialized-brain-training

~~~

Emotion: Hopeless Despair

Superman

L: I am feeling physically ill with this debilitating disease and the effects of the medication. I am exhausted, nauseous, and sometimes the vertigo is so bad it feels like the ground is moving under my feet. I don't know how I can keep up with all my responsibilities on top of my illness and my daughters' injuries. I am in way over my head and unsure I can function. When I put myself out there and tried to ask for help from others, I felt further abandoned. This must be the feeling of hopeless despair. God, is there anything you want me to remember today that could help me?

G: Remember when you were two years old and you walked into the hospital with your dad? He gave you a hug and kiss goodbye before joining your mom while she delivered your brother. You stood in the hallway with your grandma, watching him walk down the hall.

L: Yes, I can picture that. Mom was already gone, and dad was walking away. I could sense the shift in their attention.

G: Why do you think I am reminding you of this now?

L: Maybe some of my feelings are similar: hopeless despair, abandonment, unsure how I will survive. It must have felt pretty big to a two-year-old who was used to being with mom all day and both parents each night to be standing there without them.

G: Can you sense where I was in that memory and what I was doing?
~~~

L: No, I can't see you. I am beginning to worry because it's such a vulnerable place to want to see you and not be able to. All I can see are tiles on the floor.

G: It is okay. I am with you. What do you notice about the tiles?

L: They are black and white patterned tiles.

G: Yes, anything else?

L: Actually now I can see a beam of light on the floor tiles because the hospital door behind me just opened and shed a path of light on them. Somehow I see a flickering on that light path from something moving and casting shadows.

G: Intriguing. Can you keep looking?

L: Yes, it seems like somehow Jesus is standing in the door and He looks like—how awesome—He looks like Superman! His hands are resolutely placed on his hips, and He looks strong, confident, and capable. As His cape blows in the wind, the shifting shadows of light dance on the floor, creating more patterns on the floor tiles. Even though I am watching the doors ahead of me close and my dad disappearing behind them, Jesus is standing in the open doors that I am going to pass through to exit the hospital with my grandma. Somehow, because I know Jesus is strong and capable like Superman and He can handle anything, I will be able to handle it as well.

G: Yes, and isn't it great that since I am the same yesterday, today, and forever? I can still be your Superman. You can go with me and we will handle these challenges together. How does that sound?

L: Yes, I want that. I love how fitting it was for me as a two-year-old to see you as Superman.

This next conversation occurred when I was thirty-eight. I love how my intuition kicked in about breathing even before it became so popular as a tool for dealing with fear and anxiety.

Emotion: Fear

Breathing in Jesus

Despite my deep fatigue after a restless night's sleep, I woke before the alarm and noticed my four-year-old daughter and husband sleeping in the hotel room. Today was the day of her open heart surgery.

L: Oh God, I don't want to do this day. I just don't. This feels like the hardest day ever, and I just want to roll over and escape. I feel so afraid. Can overall good really come out of this day? There are too many factors for things to go wrong. The emotional strain alone could greatly impact her for life.

G: I am with you, Lisa. I will be with you throughout the day, and I will be with your daughter. The three of us have laid amazing groundwork for this day. The three of us are prepared.

L: Help me remember the groundwork, please.

Over the previous eight months, we visited countless doctors, and our daughter underwent many uncomfortable and distressing procedures. Before the completion of her supposed routine, non-invasive heart repair, we learned that her congenital heart defect was more complicated and actually required open heart surgery and intricate repair. As she struggled greatly to recover from that first procedure, we learned that her tonsils and adenoids were ninety percent blocked and required removal before the open heart surgery.

G: Remember the early morning drive to the ear, nose, and throat specialist? The doctors warned you how painful the procedure would be to have her nasal passage examined.

L: Yes, we got on the highway and saw rays of sun shining down through the clouds in vertical streams of light. She excitedly exclaimed, *"Look! God's light is shining down on us. He is showing that He is coming with us to the doctor."*

G: Remember how she processed the painful procedure with you?

L: Yes, she said, *"Mommy, when I looked at your face and saw how worried you were, it made me worry."* Oh, I was trying to be calm and reassuring, but I made it worse. I felt so terrible.

G: Yes, but consider that she was so connected with you that she read your facial expressions.

L: That is amazing for a four-year-old, isn't it? And she was so connected with herself she was able to tell me how she felt.

G: And remember that you asked her forgiveness, she forgave you and you both decided together what would help?

L: Yes, I agreed to try to keep a *"Yes"* face that conveyed *"I want us to be together even when things are hard"*.

G: Yes, and your whole family reminded each other about *"Yes"* faces.

L: A lot of good did come out of that.

G: Yes. Remember her dream?

L: Yes, I felt so relieved, comforted, and happy the morning she woke up and told us how she dreamt that Jesus took her to the zoo. They held hands as they walked, and he showed her the penguins.

G: Remember the night before she said good-bye to your parents and other daughter?

L: Yes, she was brave and strong as she led us to pray for her. She drew a picture of her chest with stitches in it, stuck it on the wall and asked each of us to slap our hand on the picture like a *"high five"* and say a prayer for her.

We settled her in the hospital room and just before we started to pray for her, they wheeled her out. I stood in the hallway, leaned on the railing, and stared outside the window.

L: I felt so distraught and helpless as they wheeled her away. She was awake enough to still lift her head and reach out to us. I feel worried that she will remember seeing us helplessly standing in the hospital hallway, getting smaller and smaller and unable to come to her.

G: Peace be with you, Lisa. Let's do this together. We will get through this. Remember how you creatively prepared her:

I had learned through years of practice that I can process trauma by understanding that God is always with us even in hard times. So I hoped that my daughters could preempt carrying unprocessed trauma into adulthood if they could sense Jesus being with them during hard times. I looked for concrete ways to instill in them the reality that even if my husband and I weren't with them, they could always rely on Jesus. We practiced like this: When we take in a big, deep breath, we think of breathing in Jesus and letting Him fill our bodies. When we blow out all our breath, we blow out all that is painful, yucky, hard, and sad and make more room for more of Jesus.

L: God, I want my younger daughter who is now in surgery and my older daughter who is ten hours away from all of us to know that you are with them no matter what.

G: That is a beautiful desire. I want that, too.

Before this third surgery, I begged and pleaded with the surgeons saying, "I am aware that this is against hospital policies, but when my daughter wakes up, I want her to see our faces. I want her to know that we are with her, and I want her to see us seeing her. During the last two recoveries from surgery, she had a very difficult time and was more distraught because she said she didn't know where we were. I don't care what we have to see. Please let us be there when she wakes up."

After praying through the surgery, they brought us into her recovery room so we could arrive before her. Seeing her vulnerable and pale body stirred an even deeper, tender compassion from my mother's heart. Watching with my own shallow breathing and tight chest, I beheld a divine moment. She opened her eyes and drew an expansive, deep breath in as her raspy, anesthesia-induced voice uttered,

"Jesus!"

L: Thank you, Jesus, that this was the first thing she said emerging from surgery and anesthesia. You were the first One she turned to, and your name was the first word she uttered. Perhaps she did not even notice us, or maybe, since she was vaguely aware of our presence, it provided the bridge for her to make *breathing in Jesus* her first action. What matters most is that she chose you and this is ingrained in her memory bank.

G: I saw her noticing you, and I heard her calling my name.

L: Please let this be the story of her life. May this be the story of all our lives, breathing in Jesus and exhaling all that gets in the way.

Disgusting physical messes are easy to identify. Sometimes, I have a hard time recognizing my disgust when it pertains to heart, soul, and relationship messes. This conversation began during a time of silent prayer in the middle of a church service.

Emotion: Disgust

The Sun/Son Is Rising on Your Soul

L: I feel cold and lonely, as if I am in a prisoner in an old basement with a damp, musty floor. My soul feels chilled. I feel disgusted by myself, situations, and people I shared my soul with. I can't listen to a favorite worship song, take communion, choreograph a worship dance, or enjoy a lot of other life-giving activities without being invaded by these painful memories and feelings of disgust.

G: I know this is pervasive and invasive for you. I know how much you are impacted by these experiences.

L: I can't improve the situations. None of my skills, resources, gifts, talents, ideas, or expertise can clean this up.

G: You have positioned yourself in a place that is giving you peace and space to listen. Do you want to remember something beautiful?

L: Yes. I definitely prefer beauty instead of disgustingness.

G: Remember when you watched the last few minutes of the Swan Lake ballet? Can you hear the music, especially the violins repeating that hopeful phrase?

L: Yes, and I see my oldest daughter so graceful, so beautiful, and so poised at such a young age. Her arms are slowly, rhythmically bending and extending as if she is a flying swan. Her strong yet quiet feet are effortlessly gliding across the floor en pointe. I am completely mesmerized by her yet able to take in the whole corps of swan dancers. I see and hear beauty that causes me to feel warm, soothed, and comforted. My disgust has dissolved.

Everything I am experiencing is appealing, and I feel reverence and admiration. Now the dancing swans are lifting their chins as they anticipate the rising of the sun. The stage lights mimic the sun rising out of the darkness and the warm glowing pinks, oranges, and yellows thaw the chill in my bones and transport me from this dark, musty basement to an expansive beach at the break of dawn.

G: The Sun is rising on your soul.

L: I feel this. The sun faithfully rises and guarantees life and warmth. The sun slowly drives out darkness one section of the planet at a time.

G: I see you turning your face toward the sun.

L: Yes, I am reminded of a science video depicting planet earth being transformed from darkness to light as it rotates toward the sun. I am here now with you turning toward *You* and feeling Your light shining onto my soul and body, one section at a time.

G: The Son is rising on your soul.

L: Yes, Jesus the Son rising on my soul. A glimmer of hope is rising in me. My desire for all of You and the True You is stirring. This is another advancement on my soul. Thank you for this promise.

As this conversation continued, I was then able to access another powerful emotion; shame. I heartily endorse the act of naming shame. Shame gets power as it hides, so I find that simply naming shame begins to dissolve it.

Emotion: Shame

I am Not Ashamed of You, Lisa.

L: For months, I have been retelling myself and others the story of the sun rising on my soul. I recount it as if I was entrapped in spiritual darkness, and as soon as I turned my face toward you and chose the real you, then the sun, Your Son, began shining on my face.

G: I know this has relieved you from disgust and brought you hope. I would like to show you something more. Do you want to see?

L: Yes. I want to see.

G: Have you considered where Jesus was?

L: I haven't thought much about that. I pretty much pictured Jesus standing in the light. When I turned toward Him during that silent moment in the church service, He shined his light on me, put His hands on my shoulders, and looked at me.

G: Jesus' hands have always been on your shoulders, and He has been looking into your eyes even when you were in the darkness. As you turned toward the sun, He turned with you.

L: Really? Wow. That is really different. I thought I had taken myself away from you. I thought I needed to repent and turn from my mistakes of chasing after false spirituality before you would shine on me, before I could feel your light. I guess I thought it wasn't until I turned towards Jesus that Jesus could be with me.

G: We have always been with you, Lisa. Jesus has always been with you even when you couldn't see. You thought you chose a spiritual path of false religiosity that I wasn't in, but I am inescapable.

L: It is hard to believe, and yet this is how David describes you in Psalm 139, isn't it?[2] I want to live like this is true. I was so confused and deceived, and I acted with pride, as if I was sure I knew I was following the True You and doing all the right things. I am so sorry.

G: I am not ashamed of you, Lisa. I have never been ashamed of you.

L: Wow. You are not ashamed of me? (long pause, lump in throat) I didn't even realize I was feeling ashamed. I guess I was ashamed of myself and certain that you were ashamed of me, too.

G: You got it. I am not ashamed of you Lisa. What if it is really not so much about making wiser choices and getting it right, but instead about wanting more of me and wanting me more?

L: That would be awesome. Jesus, I feel your hands on my shoulders, and I see you looking into my eyes. I know you are staying with me despite my mistakes and seemingly wrong turns. I want to walk through each moment of my life feeling your hands on my shoulders and seeing you looking into my eyes with love and tenderness, no matter what I do.

G: Lisa, I assure you that as you continue listening for my voice, you will hear me say again and again, *"I am not ashamed of you, Lisa."* See Jesus looking into your eyes with compassion and patience and feel His warm, steady hands always on your shoulders.

---

2. *Where can I go from your Spirit? Where can I flee from your presence? If I go up to the heavens, you are there; if I make my bed in the depths, you are there. If I rise on the wings of the dawn, if I settle on the far side of the sea, even there your hand will guide me, your right hand will hold me fast. If I say, "Surely the darkness will hide me and the light become night around me," even the darkness will not be dark to you; the night will shine like the day, for darkness is as light to you.* (Psalm 139:7-12, NIV)

L: Please take away all my shame and condemnation. I feel so responsible for my mistakes or possible mistakes and others' mistakes.

G: You are carrying a lot of heavy burdens, and I am quite happy to relieve you of them.

L: Shame is a big issue in our world and in our family. It seems like we tend to do whatever we can to resist it and fight it off.

G: I gave people shame as a gentle warning that they are veering from how I designed them. Whenever you feel a little shame, I invite you to first see me unashamed of you.

L: This reality of Jesus' hands on my shoulders, looking into my eyes and saying, *"I am not ashamed of you"*—this changes everything.

G: You can feel secure and unashamed with me no matter what you have done, then you can take the steps to act like your best, true self with others and to repair anything you are responsible for. I am with you. You can do it. With me, you can rise up from *any* situation with hope the same way your daughter was dancing like a swan at sunrise, free of all shame.

L: I am thinking of the prayer you directed Moses to have Aaron tell the Israelites. I pray that for me and us as well. *"The Lord bless you and keep you; The Lord make his face to shine upon you, and be gracious to you; The Lord lift up his countenance upon you, and give you peace."* (Numbers 6:24-26, NRSV).

Lately, I envision Jesus putting His hands on my shoulders and telling me He is not ashamed, as I simultaneously acknowledge my shame. Sometimes it seems as though He acts first and then I realize I am feeling ashamed. Naming shame is like using WD40 on a key in an old lock. The door that I struggle against and impatiently want to kick down opens effortlessly as soon as I name shame. It is as if I am releasing spiritual oil from a can and then my readiness to apologize, ask forgiveness, and act like my best self is unlocked. I like to think that old lock is on a vintage car door, and I am opening it up to hop in and embark on a road trip.

Speaking of impatiently kicking something, here are a few conversations dealing with anger that I can share without shame.

Emotion: Anger

I Want Payback (Please)

L: I feel so angry, so frustrated, and so falsely accused.

G: Who are you angry at?

L: Myself…And you, God.

G: I can handle your anger. Please tell me more.

L: I have constantly been praying for you to come through for me.

I wait.

I stay silent.

Eventually, I direct all the anger back at myself.

Right now, it feels too risky to even exist.

I am so angry, I need to take this pillow and hit it on the bed while I am crying out to you.

G: I can handle your anger, Lisa. I will always be able to handle your anger. What do you need right now?

L: I need you to come through for me. Can't you see how I am pouring myself out here trying to stay true to my conscience, myself, to justice and honor? I need some sort of payback for all this. I need relief. Please do something.

G: I hear you. It is good to see and hear you being real with me. Hang in there, Lisa. Hold on. I'm on it. You will see.

I did experience some payback a few days later and was quick to recognize and thank God for this answered prayer. It is becoming easier to recognize and effectively channel my angry energy and such a thrill to see unexpected, bountiful, and sweet fruit. Needing to spend some of my angry energy, I went for a brisk walk and had this next conversation:

I Know You Have Something More

L: I feel so angry. This new small group starts tomorrow morning and four people just dropped out. I spent a lot of extra volunteer time and emotional energy coaching and communicating with these folks, and I held the slots open for them. They just informed me they are dropping with only sixteen hours before this next class starts. I know something more is supposed to happen with this group.

G: What do you want?

L: Please give me ideas for who else I can invite to join this group.

G: What about the couple who is returning home today from the cancer treatment center? He will have to recover at home, so maybe he and his wife could participate in your online group.

L: That feels like a long shot, but I will text them.

This couple responded immediately and gladly joined the group. They asked if one other couple could join us, and we quickly became a fellowship of four couples intentionally pursuing intimacy with God, our spouses, and each other. We decided to continue meeting after the five-week course as a community of practice of leaders, and our relationships continue to deepen.

I can easily envision my less authentic self, stuffing my anger and half-heartedly limping along the course with only three people, harboring resentment toward the dropouts, and withholding whole-hearted engagement when I facilitated future groups. Instead, I now envision the life-changing potential of small groups that God prepares in advance, and I ask God first to link me up with the right people.

I have saved the strongest emotion—the one requiring the most transformation—for last.

Emotion: Sadness

Mourning into Dancing

L: I feel so much inner turmoil, confusion, and regret over some parenting decisions that still have impact today. I feel angry that I didn't have the freedom to parent and follow my intuition. I feel shut down from being a mother. How do I live from my heart and then shut down my mother's heart? My body feels half-alive, half-dead, and I am completely drained of energy. There's a lump in my throat and a pain between my eyes. I am straining just to keep my eyes open. What do you want me to remember?

G: Fourteen years ago, your daughter was sad about something that happened that day. You snuggled into bed with her and gave her a tissue for her tears. You asked her if she wanted to share her sadness with Jesus.

L: We sang *"Open the Eyes of My Heart, Lord... I Want to See You."*[3] As we sang that song, she held out her hands and showed you that she was sharing her sadness with Jesus.

G: My hands were under hers, holding them up.

L: I love that. She imagined seeing Jesus doing the jig with her, and I still treasure the picture she drew of it. You were turning her mourning into dancing like it says in Psalm 30. I love how you were speaking her language since she loved dancing.

G: I love how you stayed with her, paid attention, and gave her a safe space to feel her sadness so she could share it with you and me.

L: It is a privilege to share these sacred moments.

G: I know this was a hard day as a parent. I am proud of you for persevering. I have been proud of you throughout your life. Even though you can't crawl next to her in bed and see how she is interacting with me, rest assured that those memories and experiences are in her mind, body, and spirit, even now.

Maggie Has Trained You

Maggie was our Golden Lab/German Shepherd mix. She was sixteen years old and on her last leg. She declined very quickly, and her suffering from her probable brain tumor was increasing, rendering her non-functional. I spent three hours on the kitchen floor holding her head in my lap, waiting for the rest of my family to come home. It was clear that we needed to take her to the vet to say goodbye the next morning.

---

3. Baloche, Paul. *Open the Eyes of My Heart*. YouTube. https://www.youtube.com/watch?v=ViBNqNukgzE

Eight years prior, I was reluctant to adopt Maggie. I wasn't sure I was ready to add a dog to our lives, but I knew that my children wanted one. My oldest daughter is a compassionate caregiver, and she really wanted a dog. I saw the joy she experienced with her rabbit, so I wanted her to have that with a dog as well. My youngest daughter had some legitimate fears due to a previous experience with dogs, so I wanted to create an opportunity for joy to override fear.

The first day my husband and older daughter brought Maggie home, my younger daughter ran up and hid in her room. As she fearfully looked out her bedroom window at Maggie energetically chasing tennis balls in the backyard, I worried that we made a mistake. However, by the end of evening, she felt safe with Maggie. One time we were visiting friends, and they knew we were bringing our bunny and our dog. One child observed Maggie in the car window and said, "Is that your bunny?" because her ears were so big and stood up very tall. The other child said, "She looks like a chihuahua," even though she was quite large.

Since Maggie had won my heart, I felt very sad as I waited for my husband to come home from work and assist in bringing her to the vet to relieve her misery. I was just learning how to freely grieve, so that morning, I buried my head in her fur, wrapped my arms around her neck, and cried and cried. I told her how thankful I was for her and how much I was going to miss her. I thanked her for what she did for my family for so many years and for allowing me to say goodbye to her and to cry without holding back. Then as my husband and I sat with her in the vet's office, saying our final goodbye, I buried my head in her fur again. Knowing that her fur would no longer comfort me in my grief, I asked:

L: Jesus what are you doing right now and where are you?

G: I am standing behind you both, wrapping my arms around you both as your arms are wrapped around Maggie.

L: I feel the way you are comforting us, and I see that you are also feeling sad with us.

G: Yes. I know how much she has meant to you. Lisa, now that you have learned to freely grieve and find comfort in Maggie, you can learn to do that even more deeply with me. Maggie has trained you for this. You tried to train Maggie for years, but Maggie has actually trained you.

L: Yes, she has. Thank you for Maggie.

G: You are always welcome and invited to come and bury your head in my neck, wrap your arms around me, and grieve. I will comfort you, feel sad with you, and be with you always.

As I became more comfortable and well-acquainted with grief, it felt important to become more efficient with this emotion since it requires a lot of work and a lot of rest afterward.

Releasing Griefs of False Ideals

L: Lord, show me how to love you and follow you completely free from how I want it to be. I want to shed my false expectations, so I don't have to grieve the loss of those, too. It is hard enough to grieve real losses. I don't want to also grieve the loss of false ideals.

G: That sounds like a great idea. I will be with you as you declutter and travel lighter.

During my last few years teaching dance classes, I adopted a well-known prayer into a warm-up exercise. As we moved our bodies and looked at a construction paper cross I posted on the door, we would call out negative traits such as competition, envy, or unforgiveness, and exchange them for the opposites that could only come from Heaven, such as cooperation, honor, and forgiveness. However, I erroneously thought I could do that with my emotions as well, especially sadness. Jesus, the "man of sorrows acquainted with deepest grief" (Isaiah 53:3, NRSV) met me tenderly and helped me understand grief and sadness with more clarity.

Now Our Sorrows Are Halved

L: There is a reality to the level of pain that is being directed at me. I feel sad, really sad. Can I dance with you and bring this sadness with me?

G: Yes, you and I can be in sync with our sadness.

L: Even though I was hoping you would take my sadness away, it seems like you are just taking some of it away.

G: You are right, Lisa. I can't take away all your sadness, but I can lighten it enough so you can move forward and keep dancing.

L: This reminds me of when you said, *"Come to me, all you that are weary and are carrying heavy burdens, and I will give you rest"* (Matthew 11:28, NRSV).

G: I am feeling your sadness with you. That is what makes it feel lighter. I can't take away your sadness on this side of heaven, but I can feel it with you and be with you. That is why it feels lighter.

~~~

An important truth that accompanied my whole-hearted practice of embracing my emotions is the idea that I can choose the meaning I attach to my emotions. Feelings and truths no longer compete for the number one slot in my mind; they stand side
~~~

by side and are learning how to get along with each other. Truth speaks to feelings and sets boundaries. Boundaries, feelings, and truth are important components of the most important task we are given while on this planet: loving.

CHAPTER 6

I Have to Say I Love You in a Song

Prideful to Teachable

"Let's not pretend this is easier than it really is..." —Matthew 5:29, MSG

I have asked God a similar question many times over the past three decades. It sounds something like this:

L: There are so many good deeds that need to be done and people to help and love. Isn't it better if we all focus on that instead of our own feelings and pain?

God has answered that through many experiences over the years. Following are snippets of some of those conversations.

When I was in my mid-twenties, I worked in campus ministry. I loved being with college students, but I also heard about many painful situations and felt helpless. Learning how to recognize when I felt overwhelmed and needed rest was a skill I had yet to develop. So when my body started loudly trying to get my attention, I drove myself to the ER. After some tests, doctor visits and the recommendation to reduce my stress, I cancelled my work appointments and took a walk near the ocean. I finally angrily blurted out loud to God.

L: Here I am taking care of all these people, and now you expect me to take care of myself too?"

Busted.

L: Did I really just say that? *(I started laughing sheepishly.)*

G: Where did you get that idea? It wasn't from me. Of course I want you to take care of yourself.

L: I didn't realize that I wasn't.

G: They suggested you could learn to manage your stress by learning to recognize when you feel anxious.

L: I don't feel anxious. That's not a Christian thing to do.

The conversation ended because I stopped listening. Over the years, I finally heard and experienced God saying—

G: Do not be afraid of feeling anxious or overwhelmed. These emotions are protecting you and telling you to rest and recover so that you are caring for people out of your own health and vitality.

God had more answers to give on this topic.

G: When you are able to endure your own pain and suffering, rather than denying it, then you will have true impact loving and serving others.

This lesson came to a breaking point during my oldest daughter's junior year in college. She was dancing part-time with a company that was involved in overcoming human trafficking. I was so proud of her for applying her tender compassion for others by using her dancing to tell stories that raised awareness of the horrors of human trafficking. During one weekend, our family attended several events including dance performances and stories from speakers who had been rescued from trafficking and those who helped rescue others. These words kept ringing in my head as I listened to people and watched others dance the message:

SPEAK UP!

L: God, I can hardly bear this pain. I hate seeing people dishonored and devalued. I feel paralyzed and helpless.

G: I hate seeing people dishonored and devalued too. You are sharing my heart, but I don't intend for you to feel paralyzed. I can help you so that you can be helpful and loving toward others.

L: They keep talking about speaking up. I can't even handle speaking up effectively in my own life. How can I ever speak up for those who cannot speak for themselves?

G: You will speak up for others once you learn to handle speaking up for yourself. As you are able to stand resolute in the face of those who try to silence you, you will gain resilience to stay standing in the face of those who try to silence others. You will effectively bring honor to others when you experience that I honor you. You will effectively value others when you realize your life is valuable. When you can handle your own pain, then you can handle seeing others' pain without being consumed by it.

I created you to care about honor and value. I created you to feel the pain of dishonor and shame. Let's work together to endure this pain so you can be one who brings honor instead of shame.[1]

The Glory Realm

In September 2014, I entered another new season full of transitions and losses. To inaugurate the new season and focus on the positive, I simultaneously joined others in my church on a twenty-one day fast to draw nearer to God. I followed recommended medical procedures, stayed hydrated, and received the nutrients I needed for full days of teaching dance, commuting, and preparing food that I wasn't eating for my family. I felt energized, hopeful, and highly expectant that life would only get better as I climbed to yet another peak in my relationship with God. In all honesty, I anticipated that once I reached this peak, it would become my new base camp, and my future treks would either go farther up or occasionally back to base camp but never back to the trailhead.

As I was praying one day, a scene unfolded before me, and I watched with curiosity. I envisioned a small twinkle of light in the darkness, like the first star that appears at dusk. I fully expected that

1. The Life Model refers to this as identifying our heart values by what causes pain in our hearts. "*Caring deeply can mean hurting deeply. Everyone has issues that particularly hurt or bother him or her and are the way he/she is likely to get hurt. Looking at these lifelong issues helps identify the core values for each person's unique identity.*" Coursey, Chris. *Transforming Fellowship: 19 Brain Skills That Build Joyful Community*. East Peoria, Ill.: Shepherd's House, 2016. 262.

this tiny glow would grow into a burst of light and that God would reveal something and give me great clarity and insight. Something similar happened a few months previous, so this seemed like a reasonable expectation. I would have saved myself some heartache if I remembered (from reading Old Testament narratives, stories of Jesus in the gospels, and the adventures of the apostles in Acts) that God is too creative and desirous of a relationship with us to ever do the same thing twice.

Instead of the light increasing, dark storm clouds rolled in, almost completely engulfing the light, leaving just a spark of brightness. It reminded me of the tale of "Peter Pan," when the fairy Tinkerbell lay dying and the twinkling light that represented her life rapidly dimmed. Strangely enough, I didn't freak out or assume that I had stumbled into dangerous spiritual territory, nor did I numb out by turning to a distraction and giving up prayer. I credit myself for staying engaged with God and hesitantly asking Him a question, even though I wondered if I would sense a response from Him.

L: What was that God?

G: The glory realm.

L: The glory realm?

Honestly, I was thrilled that I actually stayed present with God, asked a question, and apparently heard something back. I wanted to know more about the glory realm and have a tangible representation of it. So while attending a conference, I sought out an artist and described the twinkle of light in the sky. I didn't tell her about the storm clouds or the words I sensed God saying. She pulled out a painting that was indeed named, The Glory Realm. Again, I was amazed that the painting she picked had the words I had heard. I loved the bright blue background, the big burst of light, the ethereal angels circling around the light, and the soft pastels around the edges that evoked memories of a soft sunset.

Several months later, after things became very difficult with many of my relationships, I came to terms with the reality that I wasn't experiencing much love or fruit of the spirit in my life or in the lives around me. I drew the brilliant conclusion that I wasn't exactly living in the glory realm. It didn't seem very much like heaven on earth. So I decided to ask another question.

What Are Those Dark Storm Clouds Anyway?

L: I know I have been quite slow on this, and in fact it has taken me several months to ask you, but what were those dark storm clouds that covered up the light?

He answered by leading me to a book titled, Joy Starts Here,[2] which used the exact same phrase. I consider this phrase in the book as His direct answer to me:

G: The dark storm clouds are relationships that need maturity, growth, and repair.

L: That makes sense.

G: Lisa, despite whatever spiritual wisdom, knowledge, expertise, experience, and training you and others have in spiritual matters, if they are not applied with love and maturity, my glory realm will remain covered by dark storm clouds.

L: I understand. This is sobering.

G: It is, but we can get through this. Are you ready to learn with me?

---

2. Wilder, James, Ed Khouri, Chris Coursey, and Sheila Sutton. *Joy Starts Here: The Transformation Zone*. East Peoria, Ill: Shepherd's House, 2013.

L: Yes. I want to learn to love. I want to see the glory realm. I want to see your kingdom come and your will be done on earth as it is in Heaven. I want to see your light shine and not be eclipsed by weak relationships.

G: Yes, I know you asked me a few months ago, when you read that particular obituary, to teach you to love.

L: Oh, I remember that, too. Is this the answer to that prayer?

G: Well, they say I work in mysterious ways.

L: Yes. Thank you for warning me, for alerting me to the storm clouds even though it took me so long to ask about them. Thank you for speaking to me and leading me to that book. I feel hopeful that you will lead me in the next steps.

G: I feel tender and concerned for you, but please know that you can change. I will stay with you, cheer you on, and coach you. You can count on me, and you can count on your brain to adapt and to think new thoughts.

L: Please show me the way. Without love, Paul says I am only a *"noisy gong or a clanging cymbal"* (1 Corinthians 13:1, NRSV). Please show me what love looks like in each situation in my life.

My brokenhearted yearning to grow in love continued, and I delved into a new phase of learning, which integrated Christian spirituality and brain science. Whenever I felt concerned for someone I loved or disconnected from them, it became a common practice to ask God to remind me of previous times with that person.

L: Could you please help me remember a time when my daughter sensed how much you loved her?

G: Remember how you all sang that song *"Good, Good Father"* frequently in church?

L: Yes, it seemed to penetrate our souls. The lyrics reminded me of a lullaby, and it was easy to waltz to.

G: Remember when she told you how she went into the school bathroom, and I seemed to surround her with my love, remind her of that song, and cause her to pause?

L: Yes, that was such a beautiful story. It really seemed to take root in her that day that you are her good, good Father.

What if every time we went to a restroom for whatever reason—to manage our insecurities, to avoid something/someone, or to use it—we stopped, felt surrounded by God, and heard Him telling us, "I am your good, good Father"? What if God is just as good whether we feel happy or sad?

We Can Handle Sadness Together

L: This is a tough day. I mainly feel hopeless despair. What do you want me to remember?

G: Well, remember when you sang that Chris Tomlin song over and over in the car and around the house, "*All of you is more than enough for all of me. For every hurt and every need. You satisfy me with your love, and all I have in you is more than enough.*"

L: Yes, that was one of many songs that I would sing repeatedly. But something is not quite right. I may have sung the words, but I am not sure I really believe them.

G: I am so glad you told me. Would you like to believe them?

L: Yes, that is probably why I sing it so much. Somehow I want to pound it into my brain.

G: Well, may I suggest that you take a gentler approach? Do you think you could identify what thoughts or emotions might be preventing you from living like those words are true for you?

L: Well, that feels big. I don't know if I can figure this out.

G: It is okay. Feel free to relax and take your time. I am here with you, and I have time.

L: I've got it! I feel afraid.

G: Please tell me more.

L: I am afraid that if I fully embrace you and let you fully embrace me, there will be no one else in my life. If I am satisfied with your love and you are more than enough then does that mean there is no one else really in my life? What if I am lonely for face-to-face connections with humans? I mean, for two years I have chosen you over anyone else and it has isolated me. I felt lonely, confused, frustrated, angry, and falsely accused.

G: So you have experienced isolation and loneliness as a result of choosing to be close to me?

L: Well, yes and no. It seems complicated. Should choosing you mean I am left alone and feeling rejected by those I thought were also choosing you?

G: Lisa, that is not how I intended it to be. I am sorry it has been like that for you. I didn't intend for my church; my body, my hands, and feet to falsely accuse, reject, and isolate others, but I did intend to give everyone the freedom to choose how they would act. My heart grieves with your heart. I died to bear those griefs and sorrows so you would not feel so overcome by them.

L: I see you with your hands on my shoulders, looking into my eyes.

G: Believe me, Lisa. I've got you. Even when you are "*worn out from [your] groaning [and] all night long [you] flood [your] bed with weeping and drench [your] couch with tears, I am with you*" (Psalm 6:6, NIV).

L: I didn't know that I could still feel so sad and still have you.

G: It is unfortunate when people think I zap away sadness like a magic trick. It is an emotion I gave you. Your mission, should you choose to accept it, is to learn how to feel it. Let me be with you and comfort you and show you how to give it its proper place in your life, no more and no less than needed.

L: Ahh, that feels like a tough mission.

G: What would it take for you to be satisfied with me being more than enough for you, even if you feel sad and sometimes despairing?

L: Wow, that is a good question to ponder.

G: I believe you can do it. What do you think is making it difficult?

L: Somehow I have a distorted way of thinking. It seems as though I can't distinguish between loving you and loving others. I can't grasp whom to love or how to love them.

G: I am so glad that you see the need to distinguish me from others. That is important. It is also important to keep asking me to teach you to love in every situation with every person. We can figure this out.

L: I want that. I want you, not formulas, and I am willing to deal with the uncertainty because I am with you.

How do we deal with the uncertainty of relationships with the certainty of God's faithful love? How do we embrace, appreciate, and seek after places of community where we are known and needed, yet still hold them lightly?

Measuring How I Am Loved

L: I am not really sure what I need, but I just want to enjoy talking with you. Could you please surprise me with a memory today?

G: Remember when you were seven months pregnant and you moved from the seminary apartments into a townhouse? You had a big cookout for all the friends who helped you move and paint your townhouse.

L: That was amazing. We had all these friends who gave their time so cheerfully. We had only known most of them for a few years or less. There was such a strong sense of belonging and community.

G: Why do you think I reminded you of this today?

L: Actually, now that I think about it, I feel isolated, lonely, and vulnerable. I have so much work to do to move out of this house, and it is so difficult to find reliable people to hire, to say nothing of friends to share the load.

G: I know how alienating this is for you. I still love you just as much as always even though you aren't surrounded by people.

L: I am remembering when you said, *"I have loved you with an everlasting love"* (Jeremiah 31:3). That brings so much hope. I want to feel held and comforted by you. I want to experience you alone as my safe place of refuge where I am loved.

G: I want that, too.

L: Please help me connect that memory and that season of my life with my present and future.

G: Back when you were pregnant, finishing seminary, and loving on your toddler, I sustained you with people. I knew you needed that. I was preparing you so that eventually you could be sustained by me first and foremost.

L: I want to remember that people are a gift from you. They can only be your hand or foot in a small way for a slice of time. They are not you.

G: There is no one like me. That is why I am called holy.

L: Yes, as much as we want to be like you, we will never be you. As much as I want others to be like you, they will never be you.

G: My love is different. It is not measured by the sum total of who is in your life.

L: I was feeling ashamed of myself for not being surrounded by helpful friends and reliable workers. I was judging myself as a failure.

G: I am not ashamed of you, Lisa. You are not a failure. Any help, any connection, any kindness from people is a gift.

L: Maybe it is okay and actually realistic not to expect it. It helps me feel super grateful when I do receive those gifts.

G: I know. Every time you naturally and joyfully appreciate that customer service person on the phone or the worker that comes to your house, you stop them in their tracks with validation, peace, and joy.

L: Yeah, I can tell sometimes they don't know what to do with my exuberance.

G: I see how their hearts are warmed as you share my love in that little slice of time. Now that you have shaken off the shame, feel free to appreciate me for who I am, and the people you do interact with for who they are. Let's stay in touch and see how it goes.

L: Yes!

We did it! We sold our house and experienced marvelous miracles seeing God provide just the right people in just the nick of time to vacate our house. There was actually more fun and adventure in the whole crazy process because I kept asking God for help and paying attention to whom He was providing. I made new friends, became reacquainted with old ones, and felt cared for by people who really cared. Quality is better than quantity!

Living without a home for five months helped me interact with the following passage in all new ways: "Then Christ will make his home in your hearts as you trust in him. Your roots will grow down into God's love and keep you strong" (Ephesians 3:17, NLT).

Where Are My Roots?

L: I feel tender and vulnerable as I think about my roots. I uprooted from my home of sixteen years where I raised my family and created many joyful experiences of love, belonging, fun, and laughter. I do believe the good times outweighed the significant hard times there. My body feels weak and inefficient, like I can't rely on it to do what I need. I want to just sit and rest and get nourished, but with this home gone and my daughters in other states pursuing their dreams, there is no soil to sink my roots into. I need to experience my roots going deep into the soil of your love instead of waiting for a home to be my soil.

G: I am delighted to be your home. Dig in!

L: I will.

G: Now, one of the ways I invite you to do that is to reach out to that kindred spirit friend. She is the right person at the right time for you. Ask her if she wants to establish a mutual time to listen to each other and me and to appreciate the memories I have given you both.

L: That sounds grand. Thank you for bringing her into my life and highlighting her to me. I will reach out to her today.

~~~

With the security of knowing that God is superior to anyone else and a good and trustworthy heavenly parent, it becomes easy and natural to ask Him for help. This is another important growth step I embark on in the next chapter.
~~~

CHAPTER 7

Ain't Too Proud to Beg

From Self-Sufficient to Vulnerable

"Embracing what God does for you is the best thing you can do for Him." —Romans 12:1, MSG

As my foundation of trust with God was being restored, I began asking for help in new ways. Rather than asking Him to change or fix my circumstances, I started to ask myself, *"If my circumstances don't change the way I want them to, or even if they get worse, what do I need in order to find joy, peace, and purpose in my life today, no matter what?"*

Once I complete the hard work of identifying what I truly need, I continue to work at staying relaxed while enduring vulnerability as I ask Him for help and wait for Him to provide. Since I agreed to partner with Him in transforming and healing me, I believe He collaborates with my brain, sparks memories, and sings songs to me. One day He lightened things up by reminding me of the song, *"Ain't Too Proud to Beg"* by the Temptations. I pulled up the song on YouTube and essentially focused on that one line while appreciating the cheerful, upbeat music. Now, whenever the song seems to randomly pop in my head, I pay attention. I stop and ask God, *"Is there something I need help with that I am not even aware of? Please help me realize what I need, so I can ask you for it."*

Since I learned that mature adults are able to identify what we need and want, ask for it, and negotiate with others, I determined to learn how to do this with God. What great training for negotiating my desires and needs with other adults.

~~~

This first interaction inaugurated a heartfelt practice of allowing myself to be more vulnerable without feeling so anxious.

Papa, Help Me!

L: Well, after two frustrating years of asking you to magically disperse those dark clouds and dissolve my pain, I have learned more about asking you for the resources I need to be more resilient.

G: Yes, I have heard your cries, especially that I would direct your heart into [my] *"love and Christ's perseverance"* (2 Thessalonians 3:5, NIV).

L: Honestly, my fear of standing before you, vulnerable and anxious and hearing silence, is still an obstacle.

G: How can I help?
~~~

L: It would help to have a tangible image of a parent helping a child when they asked.

G: How about the movie version of The Little Princess?

L: Oh, how I loved watching that movie with my daughters. The little girl who lost her spot in a private boarding school was essentially relegated to slavery when the school headmaster thought she was orphaned. The cruel headmaster called the police, who were just about to capture her when she snuck into the house next to the school where her blind father was recovering from a war injury. I can hear her sweet voice and English accent crying out *"Papa!"* as she ran into his arms, and he claimed her as his own beloved daughter. She desperately called to him for help, and he rescued her. May I call out to you, *"Papa, help me?"*

G: Always, anytime, and anywhere. I am always your *"ever present help in trouble"* (Psalm 46:1, NIV).

L: I will practice that phrase, *"Papa, help me."* So it rolls off my lips whenever I feel the first sign of fear or anxiety.

G: I want you to experience how quickly I am there for you.

L: Could you please remind me of a time when my dad was there for me—when I cried out to him for help?

G: One windy, spring day when you were five years old, your dad took you out to an open field, sent a kite soaring high up in the sky, and handed you the kite strings to fly it all by yourself.

L: Yes, I felt so strong, confident, and excited to see the colorful, dancing kite and to know that I was keeping it up there by holding tight to the kite string, until a stronger wind came up and the spool rapidly unraveled. I screamed, *"Daddy, help me,"* as I panicked that I would lose the kite forever.

G: He rushed over, grabbed the spool, wound the strings back up, and handed it to you.

L: He was so fast, and my fear changed to joy so quickly.

G: I want to help you like that, whenever you ask.

L: I want that too. What about my mom? Can you remind me of a time when she was there for me when I needed help?

G: Remember the challenges of being thirteen?

L: Who doesn't?

G: Right. One day you came home from school and felt so unmotivated and listless. Even though it was a beautiful afternoon and you were usually always on the go, you slumped down on the couch in the dark room and became sullen and lifeless.

L: Yes, and my mom, who is also always on the go, sat at the other end of the couch, looked at me and said, *"Sometimes we just feel blah, don't we?"* It was just what I needed to have her understand what I was feeling, to slow down and be with me, and give me permission to be *"low energy and unproductive."*

G: I loved watching you both resting together and totally okay with how you were feeling.

L: I couldn't even put into words that I needed that, but she knew me and knew enough about how life works to help me just by being calm and soft with me.

G: Yes, and I also want to help you like that, even when you don't ask.

L: My ever-present help in trouble, right?

G: Yes, even thirteen-year-old *"blahs"* trouble.

As mentioned in chapter one, I love knowing that I can read something in the Bible and ask God to help me understand it. Often,

I comprehend more deeply when the answer comes over time or in the midst of living instead of when I sit in front of a book or computer and drive my left brain to come up with an immediate answer.

Ask for the Ancient Paths

One afternoon, I sat on my bedroom floor, thumbing through a stack of cards I had purchased, looking for a particular card. I was interrupted from my task when a Bible verse from the book of Jeremiah jumped out at me from a beautiful card depicting a massive stone door with a Celtic cross etched in it. The door was in the middle of a bright green, expansive meadow with a worn, grass path in the distance:

"Stand at the crossroads and look; ask for the ancient paths, ask where the good way is, and walk in it, and you will find rest for your souls" (Jeremiah 6:16, NIV).

L: What are the ancient paths, God? Where is the good way? I am asking you right now for them. I don't even want to come up with my own ideas about what the ancient paths might be, and I am done trying to figure it out. All I know is that the path I am on now isn't working. I don't see our diligent efforts and energy creating much rest for our souls or the people we are trying to love. I don't know where to begin except to ask you for the ancient path.

Approximately a year later, during leadership training, a man referenced a book with the word "ancient" in the title. It triggered my memory of praying on my bedroom floor. This man relayed how, when returning to a country he used to live and work in, he made a special effort to visit a man with whom he had a falling out. He sat at the kitchen table in this man's house, looked him in the eyes, and told him he loved him as a brother. Somehow, as I listened to that simple story, I sensed God saying:

G: Lisa, this is the ancient path.

Living and loving, simply and compassionately.

Being with people and loving them.

Returning and repairing what was broken even if you can't figure it all out.

L: My heart feels captivated and stilled right now. Can you please show me what you are doing in my life in this moment?

G: Lisa, I am stretching out my arms across time from your past to your present. One of my hands rests on your shoulder where you are sitting on your bedroom floor asking me for the ancient path. My other hand rests on your shoulder now in this present moment with this small group. I am showing you a glimpse of what the ancient path is through the story you are hearing. I am stretching out my arms, the same arms that I willingly stretched out and allowed to be violently nailed to the cross. This is the same thing at work here with these outstretched hands. I am looking at your past and connecting it with your present to give you hope for the future. When you ask for something now, I will put one hand with you here. I will stretch the other one into your future to where you will see it answered, and I will accomplish another redemptive work. It is the same application of the work I accomplished on the cross for you, Lisa, and for all humans throughout history. Yes, ask for the ancient path, walk in it, and you will find rest for your soul.

Hands Like That

L: I feel burdened with concern for my daughter and confused about what to do, what to think, how to act, and who to be for her. My body is like a tightly-wound top with accumulated energy to release, but I am spinning in circles without productivity. What do you want me to remember today?

G: Remember your first summer in Mississippi with Ballet Magnificat? When your daughters were eleven and fourteen, all three of you participated in the summer dance camp. They were dancing eight hours a day and you were observing, learning, and dancing yourself.

L: That was a glorious time. My daughters felt so validated as dancers, followers of you, and as homeschoolers. They felt such belonging, such fulfillment and satisfaction. At the same time, they were stretched to choose what they believed about you and to choose whether they would trust you and become more intimate with you.

G: I loved watching them dance, making new friends, worshiping in evening services, and interacting with me. I loved watching each one of them open their hearts to me in unique and important ways.

L: I felt so relieved, joyful, and peaceful knowing that they were in your care, and grateful for other mentors who were demonstrating their love for you, commitment to become their best selves, and devotion to be excellent dancers. One daughter said she realized in a whole new way how big you are and decided she wanted to trust you with her whole self. The other one shared how she overcame feelings of shame and vulnerability in order to take steps closer to you. Then there was that incredible story you displayed before her eyes.

G: Yes, she was interacting with me in prayer, and I showed her a picture of being on a cross awaiting crucifixion. She was filled with extreme fear and dread. Just as the nails were going to come into her hands, my son, Jesus, came and took her place on the cross.

L: As she told me that story, I felt so peaceful, warm, and relaxed. I could feel the relief she felt when you rescued her from crucifixion. It was deeply validating, satisfying, and comforting to be assured as a mother that she was realizing what you have done for her.

G: I loved seeing her absorb that reality into her heart, mind, and body.

L: Not only did she share it with me, but she eventually shared it with the whole group during the sharing time on the last day of the camp. Her spunky, petite, eleven-year-old body stood before fellow dancers, company members, and teachers as she spoke into the microphone and told her story. People were weeping and smiling. Later, her counselor said, "*This morning I was asking God to show me a new way to understand what He accomplished on the cross, and God answered that prayer through her story.*" I am so glad this is part of her story, and I am so glad that your (using my seminary words) 'substitutionary work on the cross' is real. I feel so grateful. Could you please help me see what you were doing that day as she was sharing that story?

G: Oh, yes, I am so glad you asked. I was dancing, galloping, and going around the crowd, stirring them up to cheer and wave and celebrate. I was celebrating like a mascot at a sporting event, getting people to cheer, clap, stand to their feet, and initiate a wave. I was inviting everyone—friends, teachers, and dancers—who were listening to her story to celebrate what your daughter was experiencing about my work on the cross and the freedom that I give.

L: How do I connect that with my current life now?

G: I am still enthusiastically inviting people to celebrate this story. I am still weaving around your daughter and the friends, dancers, and teachers that surround her now. I am still celebrating what she and others have experienced about the redemption I offer. I am stirring them to rise up and become all that I have created them to be. I am calling forth from her the story that only she can tell in her own beautiful, unique way that will help make me real to others. I am celebrating who she was, who she is, and who she is becoming.

L: I am captivated by the movement of your hands. Is there anything else you want me to understand about that?

G: My hands are no longer nailed to the cross. They are not restricted in any way. They are not burdened. I do not carry burdens the way you do. My hands are free to wave and make circles and call forth energy, celebration, and praise from any crowd of people.

L: I want hands like that. Your hands accomplished all that I could not, but if I put my hands in yours, could I learn to move them freely and invite celebration with them as well?

G: Sure. I wonder what would happen if you focused on my hands rather than what you are carrying.

L: Could my hands become like your hands?

G: Absolutely, let's discover how well you can be the hands and feet of Jesus.

Memories, concerns, questions, quietness, and connections collaborate together in this next series. The first conversation began in a light-hearted leadership development meeting, resumed in the middle of a very difficult night, crescendoing two years later in a college baccalaureate service.

The Glistening

L: What memory do you have for me to appreciate today?

G: Remember when you, your husband, and friends left the house at 3:00 a.m. one brisk winter morning in Maine and drove three hours to cross-country ski in Acadia National Park?

L: That was an adventure. We were always doing something crazy outdoors. I loved it.

My favorite part was when I was utterly surprised by the glistening.

G: The glistening?

L: Yes, I have given this memory that title. We started skiing on the road, surrounded by big pine trees, and the conditions were not great. It was a grey day and of course very cold. I was adjusting my expectations, thinking, *It's not as beautiful as I hoped, but I will enjoy it and make the most of it.* Then we rounded a corner, the trees parted, and the ocean exploded in front of us. The open water multiplied each sparkling sunbeam, and the accumulation of snow and ice over granite added to the glorious glistening.

G: I loved seeing the surprise on your face and the way you took a break from skiing hard to slow down, breathe deeply, and take in all the beauty.

L: Yes, and I love how you blew my expectations out of the water.

G: That is the kind of God I am.

L: But you know, now I am remembering how hard things became later that night once we got home and had trouble with broken pipes and arguments.

G: There were highs and lows that day, weren't there?

I have learned that if I have a hard time focusing on a peaceful, joyful memory and my attention shifts to something painful, then I might need to further investigate what else I need to see from God's perspective. However, it is vitally important that I stay grounded in joy, peace, and strength, closely connected to God as we investigate the painful aspect of the memory. Whenever I begin to lose that connection, I set the painful memory aside, breathe deep, and then zoom in on the happy memory until God and I can walk together toward the painful "blip" on my radar.

L: Is there something else you want me to know or remember about that day skiing?

G: Actually, would you be willing to remember another ski trip?

L: Sure.

G: When you were in sixth grade, your family and another family went on a special three-day ski weekend.

L: Yes, that was very special to go overnight and ski for three days and to be around friends.

G: At one point, you were all skiing together, and you came to a little hill through a narrow wooded path. Everyone easily maneuvered down the path and then watched and waited for you.

L: Yeah, actually, I had a love-hate thing with downhill skiing at that stage. I loved the idea of skiing, but became very frustrated at myself when I felt afraid and when I was the least-skilled skier. I remember that I felt grumpy that morning, which was exacerbated by everyone looking at me and waiting for me. I was afraid of not only falling on the steep, narrow slope but also crashing into trees.

G: Can you see where I am when you were on top of that little hill?

L: Hmmm, I sense that you are at the bottom. You are smiling, waving, and saying, *"Come on, Lisa. It's not that bad. You can do it. It's going to be great."*

G: Do you remember what you did next?

L: Yes, I remember that once I started skiing down that hill, I had more fun than I could have imagined, and I did better than I thought I was going to.

G: See me at the bottom of the mountain saying, "Come on, try it. It's going to be okay. In fact, it's going to be better than you can imagine.

L: Why am I remembering this now?

G: What are you feeling in your heart right now?

L: Summer break is coming soon and our family will re-adjust to everyone being together in the house again. Normally, I would be absolutely thrilled and glad to restore our lives to their most joyful moments. But honestly, I feel fear and dread. Instead of laughter, fun, and conversation, I am afraid I am going to be put on the spot, fall, and fail with everyone standing ahead of me, watching and waiting.

G: Can you picture me calling out to you now just like I did on the mountain saying, *"Come on. It's going to be great—so much better than you think. You can handle this adventure, and you will actually have fun."*

L: Yes, I can sense that. I can believe you. I feel lighter and more hopeful. Okay, I am willing to shake off the sixth-grade grumpiness and see you ahead of me on this adventure.

G: Great! Can you imagine it will be as glorious as that winter morning in Acadia when you turned the corner and discovered *The Glistening*?

L: Oh, that would be incredible. I would love to imagine that and trust you for that.

G: Great. I am so glad we had this long visit.

A month later, the summer was exceedingly worse than I could have imagined. I felt rejection and astonishment at how readily others could betray my confidence and dismiss my concerns about spiritual and emotional abuse. I had never experienced untrustworthiness, divisiveness, and plain old meanness to this extent, especially from spiritual leaders. I grieved like there had been a death, as it tore our family apart. As this reality unfolded between my husband and I, we agreed in desperation to practice our relaxation skills for our bodies, focus our minds on something to appreciate, and then ask God:

L: What do I need to know right now?

G: It is going to be okay.

L: What? That is inconceivable. This scenario is far worse than I ever imagined. In fact, this fits in the top ten worst situations of my life. It is completely illogical to think that this is going to be okay. But you know, somehow I believe you. I feel peace and relief, which is difficult to explain. Is this your *"peace, which exceeds anything we can understand and will guard (our) hearts and minds as (we) live in Christ Jesus"* (Philippians 4:7, NLT)?

G: Yes, I am so happy to see you experiencing this.

L: My husband and I are about to tell each other what we sense that you are saying. How do I convey this to him?

G: Well, all you can do is be yourself. Remember, when you take the risk of speaking up, you have no guarantee of the response.

After our time of sharing:

L: ...Well, that didn't go so well. I actually feel more alone and misunderstood, but underneath all that, I still feel your peace. When you said this summer was going to be great, I was expecting circumstances to get better, not worse. They look much worse to me right now. However, I am guessing this peace is what you had in mind when you said it would be great.

G: Hold on to me, and let that peace sink deep into your soul. You can feel peaceful even as you feel grief, despair, loneliness, and anger. I am with you always. When you remember this night, you can remember my peace and my presence and put it in the category of memories to appreciate instead of a traumatic memory.

L: Yes, I can do that.

Less than two years later, I was sitting next to my husband and daughter at her college baccalaureate service surrounded by extended family, singing one of my favorite hymns and lighting candles one by one to symbolize the light of Christ going into all the world through the graduates and their families. With deep gratitude, I said:

L: Thank you so much, God. Of all the scenarios my brain was playing out before and after that bewildering yet peaceful night, I never envisioned this one. My heart is full. My body feels warm and relaxed, yet ready to burst with joyful energy. It was beyond my radar to realize that your outstretched arms reached between that moment when you said it was going to be okay and this moment when we could celebrate and worship together. I trust you for the things in the future that I can't see now. I see one hand on our shoulders in our current challenges and your other hand outstretched and on our shoulders in beautiful, worshipful moments that are beyond my comprehension and definitions. I see you as the God who accomplishes *"infinitely more than we might ask or think"* (Ephesians 3:20, NLT).

Keep Asking for Help

I dreamt that I was in the airport with my family and extended family. I was holding a baby in my arms and giving her as much attention as I could, despite the swirl of activity and noise around me. Suddenly, the gate changed, and my family ran ahead to board the plane. I tried to keep up, but I was carrying this precious baby. I dropped my tickets, passport, ID, and other papers. Yet, I was carefully holding the baby securely in my arms while kneeling down to pick up the papers.

Family members and airline staff were telling me to hurry or I would miss the flight. I called out, "Please, help me. Would someone please help me?" I felt atypically peaceful and confident that I was doing the best I could, and I stayed calm and held the baby well. I did not absorb the panic and anxiety I was hearing from those calling me to hurry while they kept rushing on. All I knew was that I needed to ask for help.

L: I can tell you are preparing me for something more. This was quite a dream.

G: Yes, I know you are being still with me a lot, but you are also undergoing much transition. I wanted to speak to your heart even as your body needs sleep.

L: This reminds me of that line from one of my favorite psalms: *"I will praise the Lord, who counsels me; even at night my heart instructs me"* (Psalm 16:7, NIV). I thought I didn't need to hear from you in dreams now that you and I are staying connected throughout the day. But I see I have more to learn. When will I learn to never say *"never"* with you?

G: I am patient, and you are a good student. I am glad that your heart and mind are open to learning more.

L: In the dream, I saw myself stop internally and listen to your voice when you spoke over the speakers saying, *"Keep asking for help. Ask for more."*

G: I saw you continue to cry out for help. I promise I will answer that calm, confident, consistent cry for help.

L: I trust you.

G: The flight symbolizes exciting adventures ahead. The baby symbolizes the new life you are nurturing in yourself. I am proud of you for staying calm and taking good care of that precious baby. I hear your voice asking for help with expectation that you will receive what you need to make the journey, and I see the focused look in your eyes and the strength in your body and joints. You will take good care of the baby. You will receive the help you need. You will make the flight, join your family, and enjoy your great adventure.

L: I believe that. I will speak up and ask for help even as I spend my best efforts. I will stay calm and expectant of the great adventure.

~~~

I will choose adventure and ask for whatever is needed to journey well. The resilience I am gaining by remembering and seeing God's wholehearted engagement in my life is literally getting my mind out of the ditch and back on the highway. I am ready for the road trip! I hope you are feeling as excited about the discoveries I am making in the partnership between the living God and my human brain as I am. I hope that you are beginning to connect more dots in your own history with the God of all history. Join me for the next leg of the road trip where I learn more about lightening my load.
~~~

CHAPTER 8

Freeway of Love

From Protective to Adventurous

"God brings out the best in you, develops well-formed maturity in you." —Romans 12:2, MSG

For over a year, I became triggered with painful memories and felt anxious whenever I was alone in the car for more than fifteen minutes. Yet, I completely resonated with the free-spirited abandonment and ease of riding with the top down—the *"winds against our back"* as described in the Grammy award-winning song, *"Freeway of Love."* The drums are inviting motion, energy, and freedom so that, at the very least, my toes are tapping. The blaring saxophone triggers memories of my brother on sax. Fond memories of singing hymns with my husband whenever we rode in the car during our early years of marriage also arise. How ironic that God reminded me of a song about a joyride to describe the healing going on in my brain and in my relationships. I first sensed God telling me to pay attention to that song when our small group members were practicing listening to God during our lesson on authentic relationships.

~~~

The following conversations reveal more about how I shifted out of self-protective mode and generated a stream of positive memories that re-ignited my adventurous spirit.

L: What do you want me to remember today, Lord?

G: Decades ago, when you lived on a quiet street in Maine, you brought Jennifer, your campus ministry apprentice, on bike rides. Remember the first time you took her on that long bike ride along the back roads of the rural Maine countryside?

L: Yes, she was thrilled at the fun and beauty, and I really resonated with her sense of wonder. I felt joyful, exhilarated, and valuable listening to her happy exclamations. How easy it was to provide an opportunity for her to feel refreshed.

G: Can you see where I was?

L: I envision you on a tandem bike with me—just playing and laughing. Why are you reminding me of this now? What do you want me to know about this, Jesus?

G: Ministry and loving others doesn't always have to be so hard. It is really okay to enjoy yourself and bring others with you. Whenever you increase someone else's joy, you are legitimately loving your neighbor, especially if you are fond of that activity as well. Consider this your permission slip to delight in me and my creation as much as possible.

L: That sounds amazing. But oh, this is such a contrast to how my life has been. I feel so much resentment, and I have felt
~~~

such pressure all these years to make life work. I tried so hard to raise my family in an environment I didn't choose and make the best of it for them. I have worked so hard at reaching out, sharing your love, and trying to make a positive impact. Now, after all that I have invested, I feel lonely, isolated, and without community—the very thing we relocated here for. There is so much sadness and disappointment.

G: Lisa, I know your heart. I see your intentions. It has been for good. You can't yet see what is being harvested from the seeds you have sown, but I can! Are you measuring the impact of your life by what a few powerful people in a few spiritual organizations did over a short period of time?

L: That is what I am doing, isn't it? I know that this is so distorted. I've let the toxicity of the past two years define the past eighteen years of my life. Ugh! I am still soooo frustrated with how tangled this feels!

G: Please know that's not how I see it, Lisa. If you will just watch and listen to my perspective and distinguish it from your current perspective and what others are telling you, this will get untangled. Remember the freedom that I've invited you into—you said you wanted freedom—this is the journey out.

I was desperate to see the same old painful stories that kept swirling in my mind reframed with God's perspective. I wanted to feel the exhilaration of embarking on a new road in my journey, as if I was on a tandem bike with Jesus, marveling at the beautiful countryside. I had no idea where that would lead me next, but I wanted to be off the couch, out of the house, and on the road. Remember that six-hour car ride when I listened to Jesus' words in Matthew six? Here's what happened the next day.

All This in a Fence?

I woke up feeling drained, confused, and worried about many things. My husband and older daughter were leaving the next morning for a two-week trip to Asia. Although our whole family purchased our tickets ten months in advance, we were splitting up for our summer vacations. My youngest daughter relinquished the trip to continue her ballet training, and I determined several months prior that I did not have the emotional resilience to make the trip. It was one of my first decisions ever to not push through something for the sake of family, relationships, and adventure.

I felt very guilty for declining a flight we had already paid for. I hoped that somehow in the eleventh hour, there would be a reason to apply my travel insurance so I could get credit for the flight. Perhaps a change with the airlines, illness, or a natural disaster would warrant the opportunity for me to decline the flight.

I spent a long time sitting in the backyard and talking on the phone with a prayer partner. I had so many other concerns on my mind, I actually didn't talk much about the plane ticket.

When I got off the phone, I panicked about how it was already early afternoon and I hadn't made any progress on what to do about the ticket. I started to swirl around the house, running strategies and scenarios through my head, but then I just had to stop. How could I run from God on this issue when I was going to God about everything else big or small? I stood in the kitchen, stared out the window, and asked:

L: So what am I going to do about this ticket? If there is a chance of getting credit toward another flight, I should try. Should I leave for the airport at 4:00 a.m. and hope that something will happen? It will be so hard to get to the gate and then say goodbye to my husband and daughter. What if I break out in tears or have an anxiety attack?

G: See that chair in your backyard which you sat in for the past hour being still and conversing with me and your prayer partner?

L: Yes, that was a precious time.

G: What if you went back there and conversed with me again?

L: Yes, that sounds wise as well as appealing, and it looks beautiful out there. I want to follow you and not spin my wheels apart from you, but the day is zooming by and I have hardly *"done"* anything today.

G: It is a paradigm shift to *do nothing* with me so that what you end up doing is strategic, efficient, and effective, not to mention fun and relationally satisfying.

L: I get it. That chair does look inviting.

Once settled in the lawn chair on the back lawn...

L: So what should I do about this plane ticket? Should I get up insanely early and see if something will happen or just call it a big loss?

G: Do you see the patterns of the grains of wood on that fence plank?

L: What?

G: Look at that one plank right in the center where the grains of wood almost look like a rainbow.

L: Hmmm. I see. Actually, this is amazingly captivating. I can't stop staring at it.

G: Look at the plank next to it. The stain color looks quite different, and the patterns on that are swirling circles.

L: This is so intriguing. I am drawn to this like a magnet. How can this one fence have so many different patterns and colors? Why have I never seen this before?

G: Do you think you could look at other people and situations and notice what you haven't seen before?

L: Wait. What?

G: Can you appreciate the differences between you and each person I have created?

L: That sounds like an invitation.

G: Yes, it is. Could you immerse yourself in the two different Asian cultures and trust that you can handle the challenges that will come up with your family as you travel?

L: Seriously?

G: You can handle whatever challenges will come as you stay connected with me and remember this moment, remember the fence, remember what happens when you sit down and see things through my eyes.

L: You know the challenges I have been facing. Won't I be setting myself up for failure?

G: Consider the resilience you have developed these past several months. It's as if you have learned to cross a raging river by jumping from rock to rock one step at a time. Every time you navigated rejection, disappointment, and feeling misunderstood, every time you relaxed your body when you felt anxious, rested when you felt overwhelmed, grieved when you felt sad, set boundaries when you felt demanded upon, and took care of yourself when you felt spent, you came closer to crossing that river. You can do this now.

L: I have developed a lot of resilience, and I know much better how to stay connected with you.

G: Just remember the fence and remember me saying that you can handle it.

L: Even if I can handle it, I only have sixteen hours until departure and there are numerous logistical details. What if the family can no longer accommodate me?

G: What would happen if you asked them?

L: I will try my best to see the outcome. I have been captivated by this proverb: "*Lady wisdom is at home in an understanding heart—fools never even get to say hello*" (Proverbs 14:33, MSG). I want to keep an understanding heart, Lord. I believe the key is asking you continually to help me see situations the way you see them.

I overcame many obstacles, and the family members planning the trip welcomed me into the complex travel plans. Every time we experienced a new sight in a new city or met relatives, my gratitude increased. I stopped and thanked God that I was not missing out on this important experience with my family. When I faced situations I didn't think I could handle, I envisioned myself sitting on the chair in my backyard, looking at the fence and hearing God tell me I could handle it. I continually asked God to help me see my situations the way He saw them.

Now, the house has been sold and the lawn chair donated, but I have learned the value of stopping, asking, focusing all my attention in one place, and shifting my gaze to focus somewhere else. I can do this anytime, anywhere, and God can use any object He wants.

The Fence Again, a Year Later

G: Are you willing to be still and see something in a new way—through my eyes?

L: You are inviting me to do this the same way you invited me to sit down in the chair in my backyard and look at the fence, aren't you?

G: You are on to me.

L: If I hadn't responded to your invitation and courageously overcome the obstacles, I would have missed out on important experiences, adventures, and connections with my family. I kept saying on that trip, "*I am so glad I am here.*" I want to be able to say that when I find myself on the next amazing and important adventure.

G: I am glad you want that because I want that for you as well. Is there anything that you need from me?

L: I would like the self-discipline to sit down and see what you want me to see and the courage to respond to you and to work past obstacles. I would also like an adventurous spirit.

G: I am glad you asked. I am on it, and I am with you.

While in the foggy funk of transitions in community, parenting, and vocation, I sought help from a transitions coach. The insights I gained provided encouragement and energy to wipe my tears, open my heart to the Lord and people, and pull myself off the floor to venture out again.

Embracing the Achiever

L: I am tired of wasting my time fumbling around. I need, I want, *I have to do* something constructive with my life. When I try to gather people and gather around people, I feel even more alienated. I don't know where to go and who to go to. This is disorienting and so unusual. Sometimes, I am just so afraid to try because I don't want to risk being alone, accused, and isolated again. None of this sounds like me. I am not usually this self-protective and afraid of risk. This strengthsfinder assessment confirms that you created me with strengths as an achiever, strategist, and developer (of people).[1]

I don't want or need to feel ashamed that I want to do something constructive. Please show me the way, the people, and how to follow you. Please give me a satisfying purpose and sense of direction that I can run with. I will no longer feel ashamed about desiring this.

G: I love who you are, and I am so glad that you are inviting me in. I am committed to coaching you into flourishing and being all I created you to be.

L: I love quoting Psalm 139 for everyone else, but I will say this for me, too: "*I thank you, God, for making me so mysteriously complex! Everything you do is marvelously breathtaking. It simply amazes me to think about it! How thoroughly You know me, Lord! You even formed every bone in my body when You created me in the secret place, carefully, skillfully shaping me from nothing to something*" (Psalm 139:14-15, TPT).

As you told me before, I can't afford not *to do this. I can't afford not to be my best, true self.*

---

1. Rath, Tom. *Strengthsfinder 2.0*. N.Y., N.Y.: Gallup Press, 2007.

This Is NOT My Home

A month after we moved out of our home of sixteen-and-a-half years, I visited my parents and stayed in my childhood home in rural Maine on a beautiful lake while our next townhouse was being built. Appreciation and integration abounded in my brain as I reconnected with family and friends. As I experienced the mutuality of serving the community in positive ways and receiving hospitality, joy, and kindness from others, my anxiety diminished and my sense of purpose and identity rose.

One night I dreamt that I was staying with family and friends in a house. Upon walking down the stairs and entering the living room, I was met with confusion. I knew I was in a different house, but all I could see was our previous house. Staring at my roll top desk that was in its usual place against the wall, and feeling this external pressure to accept that I was standing in my home, I loudly and repeatedly said, "No this is not my house. This is not my reality. I am not here. I am somewhere new."

L: God, something deep within me knew I was in a different house. I knew I wasn't seeing clearly. It seemed like something from my past was trying to come into my present and dictate my reality and my identity. What do you want me to see more clearly?

I paid attention to my circumstances and relationships, waiting for clarity and trying to remain curious and slow to judge. While paddle boarding on the serene lake and enjoying the blues and greens of my surroundings, it seemed like God was reminding me:

G: Remember how you learned that in dreams, houses can often symbolize your body?

L: Yes. I knew I was in a new and different place with myself. Someone or something external was trying to tell me I was in the old house when I wasn't.

G: How does that connect with what is happening in your life?

L: Actually, something like that just happened a few days ago, didn't it? I felt so blindsided and paralyzed with confusion, I couldn't make sense of it.

G: Yes, you are making the connection.

L: Yes, someone was resolutely assigning motives to my actions without really knowing me. They didn't seem to understand that I was seeking to act with integrity and respect toward others. It was as if I was being told I still lived in my former house. I knew I was in a new place, acting in a new way, and being more like my true self, even if it did disrupt the status quo. Inside I said, *"No, this is not my reality. I am not who you are saying I am."* I refused to accept the overly-asserted, judgmental message from an external authority. I am still struggling to lovingly convey this on the outside, but at least I knew what was true. It is all about perspective. I want to see myself and others through your eyes so that I don't do to others what was just done to me.

G: I am proud of you for understanding who you are and for paying attention to me, the dream, and yourself. Imagine yourself playing the game 'escape room.' You are in one room with a group of people and they think they have the solution for how to solve the mystery and escape from the room. You have another idea about the way out. Hold on to yourself and speak up about your ideas, because they have validity. You have no control over whether they are heard or considered, but they belong in the world as spoken words.

L: I also want to forgive that person. I want to learn how to be patient and non-judgmental toward that person and to try to know them the same way I want to be known.

G: That is another great idea with a lot of validity!

As transitions continued both by external circumstances and ones that I initiated, I continually chose to move forward with adventure rather than retreat into self-protectiveness. Although I defined myself as a wounded extrovert, disguised as an introvert, it became even more validating and empowering to process my life with God first before others. It likely made me a better friend as well.

Another Shift

L: I can imagine stepping into something completely new. I feel hopeful and reassured. I feel strong and confident that I can handle the next new things. Help me, please. Help us.

G: I am with you. You can handle it. Remember the line from one of your favorite hymns, "*We Rest on Thee?*" "*Strong in thy strength, safe in thy keeping tender. We rest on thee and in thy name we go.*"

L: Yes, it reminds me how thirty years ago, you seemed to wake me up in the middle of the night saying those same words. I was preparing to bring college students on a retreat, and I felt nervous about all my responsibilities and new relationships. You showed me how to balance being strong, capable, reliable, and responsible while resting safe and tender in your care. I want to navigate my new season, new relationships, and clearer identity the same way.

G: Beautiful. Let's do it together.

L: I see myself living in our new home, having amazing and important family experiences, and enjoying a big hanging basket of red geraniums outside the kitchen window. I hear the song from the Disney World Carousel of Progress ride, *"There's a great big beautiful tomorrow … and it's only a dream away."* Thank you for all these details. I am feeling very grateful that I won't miss out on having them. It reminds me of the trip to Asia, feeling so relieved and happy that I courageously moved forward with you despite my fears.

G: Persevere through this time. Continually ask to see things more clearly through my eyes.

L: Please God, *"Give me your lantern and compass. Give me a map so I can find my way to the sacred mountain to the place of your Presence to enter the place of worship, meet my exuberant God, sing my thanks with a harp magnificent God, my God."* (Psalm 43:3-4, MSG).

G: I am happy to answer your prayer and to be your lantern, your compass, and map.

Recently, while on the phone with a friend, we agreed to relax, listen to God on our own for several minutes while remembering a peaceful, joyful, pain-free moment, and then talk together about our experience. Here was my conversation with God in the midst of my visit with my friend:

L: Talking with my friend has helped me access the deep distress I am feeling. I am counting on you to help me remember and see what you see. Please come through for me, and help me remember a time when I was deeply connected with you … I am not remembering anything, but I am experiencing peace, warmth, and security. I feel so relieved and held, and it is hard to put into words … Swaddled. I feel swaddled.

G: Yes.

L: I feel like a swaddled baby.

G: This is a memory of your life.

L: My life?

G: Absolutely, for the majority of your infancy you were held, treasured, noticed, and beloved.

L: This is my story. I was too young to remember, but I believe you. I feel it so strongly right now, I can fill in the gaps in my memory and record this in my brain as my story.

G: Absolutely. Please know that in addition to the family and friends who delighted in you, I am your number one fan. Can you see my smile of joy and my attentive eyes of admiration?

L: Yes, I can see it with my spiritual eyes, I can feel it in my right brain, and believe it in my left brain. I feel whole. I am making a memorial in my mind right now.

G: I am so happy for you and so proud of you.

L: I realize how much I had magnified the image of myself as a flailing, unswaddled baby during that first month in the incubator as a preemie.

G: I know, I have been with you as you have tried to reframe this and see it from my perspective. You have made lots of great steps along the way.

L: Yes, that was a big step that day I saw you, Jesus, kneeling by me, looking in my eyes and telling me, *"I am proud of you"* as the adult version of myself held the premature baby.

G: Yes, especially that day. What about today? I see you taking a big leap now.

L: Yes, I am leaping. Right now I am creating a huge memorial in my brain of myself as a baby being held, treasured, swaddled, noticed, and desired. This is yet another 'Ebenezer' a 'Rock of help' (1 Samuel 7:12, NLT). I want to live like this is true and readily return to this memory whenever I feel distressed.

G: I would like that, too. This is your story, Lisa.

Feeling like a swaddled baby is freeing me from the need to protect myself and propelling me forward to confidently take risks in relationships and vocation. Sometimes the risk is being silent or refraining from action and sometimes it is speaking up, knowing my words could be rejected or criticized. Either way, I have my secure base, my secret place, the place where I am held, noticed and seen by my loving Papa in Heaven, my redeemer, restorer, three-legged racer, and dance partner, Jesus, and Holy Spirit, my guide and leader in the unforced rhythms of grace. The following conversation sums up the shift I made in how I viewed my life, what I learned to do with God's presence and how it healed my brain.

The Superhighway of God's Presence AKA Freeway of Love

L: Could I just bask and marinate in where I already see you?

G: Of course! I designed you for that.

L: What if I can choose to focus on where I do see you instead of where I don't see you in my history. Can I just choose?

G: You are always free to choose. I hope you never force yourself to go to a painful place or allow someone else to suggest you go there. At the same time, you are also discovering that when you and I are joyful and peaceful together, we can do our three-legged walk to those places that you can't see me, and you end up discovering me.

L: Yes, and then those become the memories where I do see you. What if I looked at these moments where I saw you in my history as dots to connect in a coloring book?

G: Sounds creative. Sounds like you. Sounds like me, your Creator. Looks like you coloring on the sailboat.

L: What if I looked at these moments where I saw you in my history as stones in a river that I can leap from one to another like crossing a river?

G: Sounds fun! I already see you leaping, remember?

L: I would love to just do that rather than putting this huge demand on myself to sort through everything negative in my past, rather than letting my feet get all tangled up, tripping over myself. Why don't I just leap from stone to stone on the superhighway of your presence?

G: The Superhighway of my Presence. I like that.

L: I see myself leaping from stone to stone, from Ebenezer to Ebenezer, from positive memory to positive memory, from one strong new thought in my brain to the next.

G: I see you, too. I am cheering you on and enjoying watching you. At the same time, I am leaping beside you.

L: Yes, my memories of your presence in my life are getting my brain and my body out of the ditch of despair, anxiety and negativity as new thoughts have formed in my brain. I see them interconnected and lit up like a supernaturally glistening motherboard.

G: Yes, yes, yes!

L: The superhighway of your presence in my life is my freeway of love.

G: Let's Go!

L: We're going ridin' on a freeway of love, winds at our back!

Where Is This Road Trip Leading?

When I first began practicing the discipline of appreciating a pain-free memory for three minutes, I chose a specific place where I was outside enjoying nature. My entry for favorite place in my high school senior yearbook read, 'by the lake in back of my house.' Our family built this home in rural Maine when I was twelve years old, and thirty-three years later it still has its designated space in the parking lot of my mind. I strolled down to this idyllic resting place of pine needles and soft moss when I felt happy as well as sad, and I felt proud to bring friends there. I am so grateful for the sacrifices my parents made to raise us in a peaceful, beautiful place that allowed us to both play hard and relax well.

My list of memories to appreciate expanded and the focus was always on my interactions with God, except for memories related to my favorite place. The distinct details of what I saw, heard, and smelled, and the peace I felt in my body whenever I remembered my favorite place was unmatched by any other location in a memory. One afternoon during a counseling session where I reflected on my favorite place, it felt vitally important to say to God:

L: I need an additional favorite place that I have chosen as an adult. Could you please help me find one?

As usual, as soon as I walked outside the counselor's office, my thoughts splintered at lightning speed into several different directions. I left the building, climbed down two flights of stairs, and walked across the parking lot. So I was completely surprised when I opened the door to get in my car and God captured my attention:

G: You know how you asked for a place? I have one for you.

L: Really? That was fast. Where is it?

G: It is a place you can always get to anytime and anywhere.

L: Well, if it is near or in my house, I just don't think it will captivate me like my favorite place on the lake.

G: I know. That isn't where it is.

L: Okay, where is it? You know I am so weary with driving.

G: I sure do know, and I have seen how it has worn you down. What if a physical place was just training ground for the place you are ready for now?

L: What do you mean? I don't feel ready for anything.

G: I have heard you ask me continually over the past few years to show you how to stay in the *"secret place"* with me anytime and anywhere. What if your new adult place you are asking for is this secret place?

L: Oh my goodness. How could I have not seen that before? The two places I am asking for are really the same thing. My new, adult place of joy and peace is not tied to a specific geographical location or a memory of being in a physical place, but it is the secret place,[2] the abiding place,[3] in the shelter of the Most High.[4]

G: Yes, anytime, anywhere.

---

2. Psalm 51:6, Psalm 139:15, Isaiah 45:3 (NIV)
3. John 15:4,5 (NRSV)
4. Psalm 91:1 (NRSV)

L: I'm in. Let's go. Thank you so much for helping me see this and put it all together.

G: My pleasure, as always.

Seventeen months ago (about a week before I saw the fence and then flew to Asia), I felt utterly deflated as I sat with my family saying, "I will probably not travel much after this." We all agreed how sad that was. Tonight, as I edit this book, I am returning from a three-week solo road trip from Virginia to Nashville, Tennessee, which I made without getting trapped in negative memories.

During today's eight-hour drive, I remembered all the travel adventures I have been on. In fact, most of the work on this book was accomplished on this road trip. I have experienced God as my Good Shepherd and the pillar of cloud by day and fire by night.[5] *Only God could bring out the best in me like this. I love how God works, and I love how I work. I can be in traffic, even in long stretches of highway, without feeling anxious or lonely. I can quickly toss out painful memories and unproductive thoughts when they jump into my head, access God's loving presence, and get back to my contented, joyful frame of mind. I feel confident and grateful that my brain can continue to heal, and that every investment I make in my mental health and relationship with God is worth it.*

Three years after that meltdown in the car described in chapter one, and one week after returning from my Nashville road trip, I left our friend's house with a full car packed with belongings to move into our new home. Departing ahead of my husband, I expected

---

5. *"After leaving Sukkoth they camped at Etham on the edge of the desert. By day the Lord went ahead of them in a pillar of cloud to guide them on their way and by night in a pillar of fire to give them light, so that they could travel by day or night. Neither the pillar of cloud by day nor the pillar of fire by night left its' place in front of the people"* (Exodus 13:20-22, NIV). Instead of a roadmap, the Israelites followed a dynamic, creative, surprising God. I embrace and endorse this lifestyle and want more of it.

to beat the morning traffic around the Washington D.C. beltway. However, the traffic was so thick due to multiple accidents that I followed Waze straight through the city of D.C. during morning rush hour—something I said I would never do.

Instead of panicking in the present stressor or being triggered by past stressors, I marveled at the Washington Monument, the cherry trees, and how close the road ran to the Potomac River. At the same time, I mulled over the brilliant thoughts I was integrating from the audio version of Anatomy of the Soul,[6] *in awe of what my body and mind were capable of. Then my spirit joined the party as I sensed God saying:*

G: I have a name for your secret place.

L: Really? What is it?

G: Vitality City.

L: How perfect! I love the word vitality. It describes how I want to live: exuberant, full of power, and strength to live and grow, continuing a purposeful existence.[7]

G: It describes you, Lisa.

L: I could not have gotten to this place without you. Thank you so much!

G: My pleasure! Isn't it great to be on a road trip together—adventure, unknowns and yet you know where you are headed—Vitality City? A place for all eternity and a place for every moment of this amazing life.

~~~

6. Thompson, Curt, MD. *Anatomy of the Soul.* Carrollton, TX: Tyndale, 2010.
7. https://www.dictionary.com/browse/vitality
~~~

Keep Moving Forward

This last conversation with God is a terrific, grand finale to this chapter. Four weeks after driving to my new home, we experienced several days of unfortunate challenges. It was Monday afternoon, and despite having little sleep and stomach troubles, I felt energized by how my husband and I overcame several obstacles and found solutions to our problems. The process involved stopping when we felt overwhelmed, talking and listening to God on our own, and then talking together.

I was on the last leg of my solo two-hour drive with a car full of our belongings to bring to our new home, and I was approaching a four-and-a-half mile bridge. Driving on bridges is not my favorite thing to do. Four-and-a-half miles is pretty long for a bridge, but I resolved to deal with my fear and overactive imagination.

There are actually two three-lane bridges that connect the island to the mainland. One bridge is for eastbound traffic, and the other bridge is for westbound traffic. However, I discovered the hard way that sometimes the traffic pattern is adjusted to account for construction or commuter traffic. As I approached the tollbooth before the bridge, I decided at the last moment to veer left for the vacant tollbooth.

Suddenly, I found myself heading east on the westbound bridge. On my left, I saw two lanes of traffic heading west. On my immediate right, I saw a guard rail with open views of water and boats below as well as the eastbound bridge and three lanes of moving traffic. (Oh, why didn't I stay left and take the eastbound bridge?)

Then a flood of thoughts came. Most of these were thoughts I had never had before: This car is so old. What if it breaks down on the bridge? Is this gas gauge working? What if I run out of gas? Why is the car behind me traveling so close to me? Why isn't there a road shoulder? I am trying to do my breathing exercises, but what if I pass out from exhaling too much?

Then I began my monologue with God:

L: Please help me. Please help the car work. Please help me focus on the road ahead of me, not the cars, water, and boats on either side. Please send your angels to protect me (Psalm 91:11, TPT). Why can't I remember and recite all of Psalm 91? Our Father in heaven, holy is your name, your kingdom come your will be done. Oh why does this bridge look sooo long? Why are these guard rails more open than on the westbound bridge? … on earth as it is in heaven. Help me. I can't concentrate. How am I going to get through this?

G: Keep moving forward.

L: What?

G: You can't afford not to move forward.

L: Oh my goodness. You are talking to me even now.

G: You can do this.

L: You are reminding me what Jesus said when we were on the gray bench.

G: You are remembering.

L: There couldn't be more perfect words to hear right now. I literally have to keep moving forward.

G: You got this. Don't shrink back. Don't give up. The cost is too great.

L: I absolutely cannot afford not to do this. I can't give up. I can't turn back. I can't pull over and rest. I can't stop and create an accident.

G: You can do it. I am with you. You are stronger than you think. You can rely on me. You can rely on you. You can rely on the car.

L: Here I am blabbing away, and it didn't even occur to me to listen to you when I feel so panicked and trapped on this bridge.

G: That's okay. That's why I spoke up. I am so proud of you for hearing me even though you felt so panicked and trapped on this bridge.

L: I did it. Thank you for talking me through this.

G: You did a great job remembering what we already talked about.

L: It really mattered that we had those conversations, and that I have these words readily available in my memory bank.

G: I remember all our conversations. They are so valuable.

L: And useful for everyday life. Those words were originally about me moving forward in trusting you. Today they were just as applicable in keeping my car moving forward. I love that.

G: Me too. I love *you*!

~~~

When I reluctantly left New England and moved to Virginia eighteen years ago, I told God that if I had to move, I wanted to be sure I was swept up in a life of seeing God do what only God could do. Of course, I thought this meant impacting multitudes and accomplishing miracles. I had no idea how much I needed God to do miracles with my mind. Over time, I have realized that any accomplishments that would spread wider than me have to come out of the overflow of God's good work in my mind first.

As I became more real in my dialogue with God, my daily life changed. My anxiety and despair decreased and my vitality
~~~

returned. Now that I have learned the techniques that allow me to cruise past those emotional obstacles, I feel confident that the One who loves my soul has my back. I feel it in my mind, body, and spirit. Realistic expectations that God will share His perspective on how He sees me exist in the core of my being. I believe God is eager to help me see life through His eyes and collaborate with me on how to navigate its' complexities. God is just waiting for me to ask. When my mind begins spinning with negativity, I adeptly shift into another gear and employ the skills I have developed.

Even when I feel sad, angry, afraid, ashamed, and confused, I enjoy relaxing with God and knowing God enjoys being with me. I have seen incredible payback when I resolve to keep the conversation going even when I feel like giving up. I compare it to skillfully maneuvering a roadblock on the highway so I can stay on the journey. Together, God and I appreciate God's presence throughout my life and in my current moments. Receiving strategies, solutions, and healing of pain from God is actually a fabulous by-product of the joy of being with God and knowing God enjoys being with me.

I hope you feel intrigued about how to engage in real talk with God and how to get your head out of the ditch of despair and onto a road trip full of hope and joy. The last chapter includes anticipated questions and responses, my thoughts about Bible reading and specific ideas for how to move forward developing real talk with God.

CHAPTER 9

Questions and Responses

Did you make shifts in beliefs and mindset that made it easier to talk and listen to God?

Absolutely. Transformation requires mindset shifts. These are my top two:

1. **I am in a life-long process of seeing myself and others through God's perspective.**

   The following quotes were complete game-changers for me in understanding the real problem with me and the human race. This pertains to Adam and Eve's disobedience to God's one rule—not to eat from the tree of the knowledge of good and evil.[1] I hope I will always embrace these truths and that they will prevent me from a self-sufficient misuse of power and knowledge.

Here are a few excerpts from chapter 5 of *Living from the Heart Jesus Gave You:*[2]

When Adam and Eve set their hearts to listen to the serpent and let him direct their choices, they ate from the tree of the knowledge of good and evil. That moment they gained for us flawed discernment… Now we all have this human birth defect which Christians are used to thinking of as our "flesh." Christians are used to thinking that the "flesh" (or sark) makes us do bad things. Actually, the sark's most harmful effect is that it makes us think we are doing something right and good when we are actually doing or thinking the wrong thing. This happens each time we figure things out on our own instead of following God's direction…

Becoming a Christian and receiving the Holy Spirit does not take away the problem…

Our wounds and the slanted teachings of our well-intentioned mentors add to the confusion…

Trying to figure out if something or someone is "good" always plunges us into error. We are always wrong—wrong because we do not see all that God sees. In fact, it is only with long training that the most mature can even begin to sense what God thinks is good and evil (Hebrews 5:14). Typically, the harder we try to correct things and do things right (the harder

1. The rest of the story can be found in the Bible book of Genesis chapters two and three.

2. Friesen,, James, James Wilder, Anne Bierling, Rick Koepcke, and Maribeth Poole. *Living From the Heart Jesus Gave You*. East Peoria, Ill: Shepherd's House, 2013.

we use the sark), the farther we get from listening to our heart. We all have this birth defect...

The fight we have between this birth defect and the heart Jesus gave us never comes to an end during our lifetime...

~~~

2. **I will never get it right, therefore I must refuse to use cruise control on this road trip.**

   Getting it right is no longer one of my goals. Every time I start analyzing, rationalizing, and strategizing a way to do right and be right, I repeatedly tell myself, *"I am right with God because of Jesus. It is only and always because of Jesus."* This is what matters most. My top priority is to stay intimate with Jesus and to see what He sees. Perhaps my heartfelt interaction with the book of Romans has had the biggest impact on shifting my attitude about being right with God.

   I no longer want to strive like Phil Collins, Bill Murray's character in the movie Groundhog Day, who had to relive the same day over and over until he treated everyone right. Who has the energy for that exhausting futility? How fitting is King Solomon's description throughout Ecclesiastes as *"chasing after wind."*[3] No, I want to devote each unique day to keeping my heart in tune with God's heart. Instead of chasing after an unseen force that will always leave me in the dust, I prefer to stand firm, facing the wind as I fly a kite with my hand connected to a dancing source of joy and beauty.

   As freeing as this invitation is to live continually dependent on God for His perspective, it requires vigilance. Sometimes, I find myself trying to determine if other followers of Jesus are judging what is right and wrong with their sark (see above

3. Ecclesiastes 1:14 (NRSV)
~~~

quote) or if they are earnestly trying to see themselves and others through God's eyes. I ask God to flash a big yellow caution light when I try to figure out others' motives and actions. Every relationship requires my constant curiosity and intentional dependence on God.

Aren't you approaching God really casually? Isn't this disrespectful?

Have you noticed how the Bible is full of metaphors? I believe God also provides us with metaphors that are unique to our context, culture, and periods in history. Since God loved us enough to bring Jesus to learn our way of life, I believe God loves me enough to speak my language. So when I sense God is forgiving me, it sounds to me like, *"No worries, I forgive you."* The Old Testament talks about how God *"will delight you with his songs"* (Zephaniah 3:17, The Message). I believe that one of the ways God sings over me is by reminding me of songs that were a source of joy and inspiration at one point in my life, even if they were not specifically written about Him. I still sing and dance to those songs that are some of the chapter titles when I need to remind myself that God loves me, believes in me and is so much bigger than the box we put God in.

The more time I spend with God, the more God seems to give me permission to interact more casually. I can interact this way with God and also be in total awe of Him at the same time. I marvel at how God is so much better than me and other humans, and I understand that God really likes and loves us.

What about the Bible?

I have always prayed that I would be a person like Jeremiah when it came to God's word: *"When your words came, I ate them; they were my joy and my heart's delight, for I bear your name, LORD God Almighty*" (Jeremiah 15:16, NIV). In addition to creatively devouring God's words in the Bible, I was a wholehearted student of Bible study methods who trained others in leading Bible studies. When I went to seminary, my final thesis consisted of an integrative project answering the question, "*How can adults stay motivated and in love with God and Bible reading?*" Twenty years after completing that project, I must conclude that my motivation and love for God and the Bible are directly related to what I want to get out of my Bible reading. When I desperately want an authentic relationship with God above all else, the Bible indeed becomes "*my joy and my heart's delight.*"

How important is it to read the Bible if I am trying to listen to God directly?

After spending three decades reading and studying the Bible, there are easily accessible words, phrases, and stories that readily pop into my head as I converse with God. Because of this, I can pay better attention, make connections, and remember previous times when I have heard them. There is great value in steadily filling our memory banks with those stories, words, and phrases. Admittedly, I still have habits to strengthen in reading all of the Bible for breadth and understanding as well as for depth.

The Bible mentors and instructs me like a teacher or older sibling by giving me stories and words that validate my experience. It also assures me that I am not alone and that anyone can recover from mistakes. When I read about how Jesus loved people when he walked the planet, I understand what God is really like. Observing Jesus' perfect example of love and compassion, gives me practical ideas on how to treat people. Whether we have been reading the Bible for three weeks, three years, or thirty years, I believe the Bible is an integral tool in developing my relationship with God. I want to keep my heart and the right side of my brain engaged, even as the left side of my brain is striving to solve a problem, answer a question, or make an important connection.

This approach to life is new to me. How do I balance Bible reading with *Real Talk with God*?

I hope that people who are new to reading the Bible will read it simultaneously while talking and listening to God. Perhaps by doing this, they will avoid the untangling that many of us who overindulged the left side of our brain need to undergo. What if we asked God to explain something that is confusing to us when we are reading the Bible before we consult a footnote, commentary, sermon, or another person? For example, over the years, it has become common for me to jot down a phrase or story in the Bible and ask God, *"Would you please show me what this means in real life?"*

There are so many Bible study methods, guides, and courses out there. How do they fit into this kind of lifestyle?

It has been helpful for me to experience a form of contemplative group Bible reflection called *Lectio Divina*.[4] At first, I had to give my left brain permission to chill out and let go of the many rules I once learned about how to study and preach the Bible. Lectio Divina allows small groups of people to alternate between interacting with God silently over a few words or phrases from the Bible and then sharing what they are thinking and feeling. Facilitating small groups in this practice is one of my favorite coaching activities.

---

4. https://ocarm.org/en/content/lectio/what-lectio-divina

I made an important shift when I decided to believe that Christ is King over all things including Bible reading. I once believed that *"context is king."* Namely, I needed to understand the context of the whole book or whole chapter before I could understand what God was saying in a phrase or sentence in the Bible. God invited me to reconsider this one night, and it has had a lifelong impact on me:

Let Mutual Love Continue

When my husband and I were dating, we returned from a prayer conference and decided to practice conversing with God together each day. We agreed that we would not talk about marriage, but rather ask God if we could begin talking and praying about marriage. One time, as we were silently praying together, my husband asked God about marrying me. He said this was the first time he truly sensed God speaking to him after believing in God for over twenty years. He heard God say, *"You choose."* I noticed that he was instantly energized, as if being relieved of a huge burden. He was thrilled to hear God giving him freedom to choose. This sounds so much like God to me. (Remember chapter two?)

Since it was vitally important that I heard from God and made my own decisions, I continued asking God similar questions. One night, I woke up suddenly in the middle of the night and these words popped into my head, *"Hebrews 13:1."* I recognized this was a Bible verse, but I didn't know the words. I got out of bed and searched for my Bible, until I remembered it was in the car. Since I didn't want to retrieve it in the dark of night, I searched for a different Bible in my apartment. I found one on my shelf and read Hebrews 13:1: *"Let mutual love continue"* (NRSV).

Hmmm, that seemed like a direct encouragement from God to keep moving forward in my relationship with this man. Before I met him, I was sure I was content to be single, with God as my husband. Oh, the adventures and precious relationships I would have forfeited if I had only listened to my self-protective heart.

The next day, when I retrieved my usual Bible from the car, I looked up Hebrews 13:1, which read, *"Brothers, love one another"* (NIV). Well, if I had read *that* in the middle of the night, I am not convinced the scripture would have had the same impact on me. I wonder if my husband would have still become the father of my two incredible daughters if I dogmatically ruled out that God was answering my request for His guidance because it didn't exactly fit the broader context of that section of the Bible.

Why don't you teach more from the Bible?

Often in my conversations with God, Bible passages will come to mind. I intentionally omitted some Bible passages that were included in my conversations. This is my invitation to you to connect the dots. I hope this creates headspace for Bible verses and stories to come to your mind. I would much rather be a catalyst for you to make your own connections between mind and heart, Bible and relationship with God, and questions and answers. I hope the truths you and God discuss will be more deeply internalized.

What should I do if an idea comes to mind while I am trying to talk and listen to God, and I think it is from the Bible?

Often, phrases and stories from the Bible come to my mind as I am interacting with God. I like to search on Bible Gateway to find the verse and chapter.[5] Then I look at it in different translations to find the words that most engage my heart and read them re-

5. https://www.biblegateway.com/passage/

peatedly, including the sections just before and after the phrases that I recalled.

What are some ways God might speak to me?

Before exploring that question, may I encourage you to start with a tiny bit of faith that believes God is always with you and wants to speak to you even if you can't sense that? God speaks in a way that is unique, personal, and completely relevant to you. God invites you to dig deep and discover how He speaks to you and how He listens to you. Your perseverance and willingness to experiment, and pay attention to your process will be more than worth it. I just read this verse today and it seemed like God was once again inviting me and coaching me to not give up.

> *"Don't look for shortcuts to God. The market is flooded with surefire, easygoing formulas for a successful life that can be practiced in your spare time. Don't fall for that stuff, even though crowds of people do. The way to life—to God! —is vigorous and requires total attention." (Matthew 7:13, MSG).*

My conversations reveal many different ways that I sense God speaking. I hope they spark your curiosity and expand your imagination to consider how God might convey His thoughts and feelings. Some of the ways you have read about include songs, memories, Bible stories, phrases, words, emotions and dreams.

I continue to learn how to respond to impressions (e.g. the Glory Sheet, Jesus and Me on the Bench, I See the Race You Are Running). I have developed the practice of taking time and allowing each part of my brain, my heart, and even my body to carefully interact and respond to impressions before nurturing them and acting upon them. I often ask God to help me *"take every thought captive and make it obedient to Christ"* (2 Cor 10:5,

NIV). I need to sense that the impression aligns with what I believe about God's identity and my identity. I believe that the messages and impressions that are truly from God will continue to bring positive change in my life and relationships.[6]

I pay attention to thoughts and how I react to them: new spontaneous thoughts, persistent thoughts that won't go away, intriguing thoughts that I want to learn more about, and distracting thoughts. I also pay attention to ideas and how I react to them: Some ideas connect my reality with a new possibility (e.g. Three-Legged Dance), and some ideas seem impossible to fulfill unless I ask for God's help (e.g. keep moving forward in Simply Jesus, Okay with Grey).

Please remember these are descriptions of some of the ways I sense God speaking to me, not prescriptions for how God will speak to you.

I wonder what would happen if you asked yourself some further questions on this topic:

How much do I really desire to interact with God?

Am I staying continually open-minded to any way God might speak to me?

How do I know if it is God speaking?

One of the ways I address this common concern with coaching clients is to first have them consider a few simple questions. I hope you take a pause and jot down your response to these questions:

- Who am I when I read the Bible?
- Who am I when I pray?
- What is God like when I read the Bible?

---

6. I often ask God to help me learn from my mistakes, repair any damage done to others, receive God's forgiveness, and forgive myself whenever I have nurtured and acted on an impression that is not from Him.

- How does God relate to people, including me?
- What do I believe is true about our relationship?

I wrestled with whether I was hearing from God or not when I went through my own spiritual confusion and was recovering from spiritual abuse. You witness in this book the resolutions that my conversations with God brought forth.

Now that I am on the other side of this question, I often feel perplexed at how we trip over ourselves with this issue. How can we restore the simplicity God offered us when He gave Jesus to the world? One of the most empowering verses I often remind myself of is, *"The Spirit of God, who raised Jesus from the dead, lives in you"* (Romans 8:11, NLT). What difference does that make in my ability to hear a God who wants to be known and heard by us?

What if I erred on the side of belief? I believe God is good, merciful, loving, forgiving, gracious, compassionate, trustworthy, slow to anger, and rich in love as He is described throughout the Bible. For example: *"But you, O God, are both tender and kind, not easily angered, immense in love, and you never, never quit"* (Psalm 85:15, MSG).

So if I believe God is like that and I ask God to speak, can I trust God to speak? I love how Jesus said:

> *"For everyone who asks, receives. Everyone who seeks, finds. And to everyone who knocks, the door will be opened. You parents—if your children ask for a loaf of bread, do you give them a stone instead? Or if they ask for a fish, do you give them a snake? Of course not!" (Matthew 7:8-10, NLT).*

If I am asking God to speak, and He is the most truthful and authoritative voice in the universe, would He allow me to hear trash? Since Jesus was referring to asking for the Holy Spirit's activity in our lives in the passage above, and Jesus promised that the Holy Spirit would *"guide you into all truth"* (John 16:8), can I trust that if am asking God to speak truth and He is truth that I will hear truth?

If I am syncing my heart to God's heart, and God is shaping my heart to be like His, is it possible that I actually don't always need to figure out which one of us is speaking? I would rather spend my energy appreciating, remembering, and applying all the delightful words I am devouring. As previously mentioned, sometimes I tell God about a Bible verse I love, and other times it seems like He is reminding me. It's all good!

Sometimes I hear something that is surprising, unexpected, or completely off my radar, like many of the good memories from my life. What an invigorating experience that is, even if it results in a gentle correction. Although I am a creative person with strengths in generating many ideas quickly, God's ideas are so much better than anything I could come up with on my own that I readily attribute those surprises to God. They illicit in me a sense of joy and peace that I could not muster alone.

Although the Bible says access to God and *"every spiritual blessing in the heavenly places"* (Ephesians 1:3, NRSV) is readily available, it is very common for external factors to distort, distract, and block us from receiving them. (Remember chapter four reveals how God and I removed distortions and how significant it was when I could see myself and God clearly.) If only we could stay clearly focused on the resources God has planted inside us and who He truly is for us, perhaps we could avoid some of the confusion we allow and create for ourselves. Our task is much more significant now because so much information is completely accessible any time, day or night.

Isn't it audacious to think you could know God's thoughts and feelings?

I believe God wants to be known. That is why God sent Jesus to earth. Knowing and being known by others is hard and full of mistakes to learn and recover from. I believe God can handle my attempts and mistakes at knowing Him and being known by Him. More than that, I believe God delights in me, believes in me and cheers me on like a parent watching a child learning to walk.

Although I advocate for starting with blank journal pages, I also strongly endorse *Joyful Journey*.[7] This helpful, easy-to-use tool contains journaling exercises which empowered me to consider how God sees me, hears me, cares about my concerns, and wants to help me. It was easy to take baby steps by first sensing God saying, *"I see you wearing your red sweater, writing in your journal, sipping your Earl Grey tea, and wiping your tears."*

I am reacting negatively and feeling stuck. What next?

When I have a strong and negative reaction I now ask myself, am I trying to avoid feeling pain that I actually might be able to handle if I used a different approach?

Several years ago, I listened to a lecture by an author and speaker who endured a traumatic experience that impacted her whole family. Paralyzed by her painful narrative, I shifted into what I call *"left brain mode."* My analysis included questioning her content and credibility as a speaker, and making a mental list of the philosophical and theological reasons why I could not agree with her. Next, I formulated strategies with my family so the same situation would never happen with us. In retrospect, I wonder how often I prevented emotional growth because I did not have

---

7. Wilder, James, Anna Kang, John Loppnow, and Sungshim Loppnow. *Joyful Journey*. East Peoria, Ill.: Shepherd's House, 2015.

the emotional capacity to feel tender toward others when they were in painful situations or the resilience to accept that life can be arduous and uncontrollable.

Now although I shared minimal details about my specific traumas, it is still possible that you might want to shift into your own left brain mode as you hear me talk with God about my pain.

Here are some techniques I use when I notice my left brain overreacting. I take a few deep breaths, notice tense muscles in my body, and yawn a few times. Then I identify some feeling words and write them down. I read them out loud and literally say, *"God I am feeling ..."* Then I ask God, *"Is there anything you want me to see about my reactions that I am not seeing clearly?"* Sometimes I keep a page in my journal specifically for analytical questions. I imagine myself putting them in this mental file and shutting the drawer, knowing that God and I can return to them after we interact heart-to-heart.

I have always been commended for being a good listener. As people openly shared personal challenges, I listened sympathetically, maintained eye contact, and sincerely demonstrated appropriate nonverbal communication. However, if I became too overwhelmed, I shifted into left-brain mode again. My slick coping techniques involved categorizing helpful resources in my mind and then suggesting books, workshops, conferences, organizations, and churches. Perhaps I came across as a cheerful walking search engine, but I wonder how much of a genuine relationship was lost because of my disguised form of emotional detachment.

Now that I have increased my resilience to pain, I feel much more satisfied when I stay in the present moment with people. I have learned that quality relationships require us to activate every part of our brain. The right side of my brain says, *"Pay attention to your emotions and the physical sensations in your body."* The left side of my brain says, *"Put words to those feelings, hear yourself speaking them, and make logical connections between what you are hearing, saying, and feeling."*

Now if you and I were discussing life's challenges, I would stay fully engaged, listen, and reflect back your concerns, as well as share some of my own. I would ask if we wanted to invite God to explain how He sees our situations. We would likely acquire new ideas and gently relinquish unhelpful attitudes, beliefs, and behaviors. I have learned that relationships are much more satisfying and sustainable when we listen well, validate each other's experiences, refrain from giving unsolicited advice, and invite God into the conversation. So rather than steer us off course by talking about resources, I would wait until the end of our visit to ask if I might offer a suggestion of resources that might be helpful.

As a diligent student, avid learner, and health geek, I have turned much of the valuable information from many well-trained and well-researched authorities into skills and habits. However, I took a lot of detours from forming habits because I was too busy chasing after more books, conferences, and online resources. Once my fuel tank was on empty and I felt too anxious to attend another conference, I started relying on myself and God to implement internal changes. So if you are feeling stuck, please ensure that you are not chasing after a left-brain detour, leaving your heart and the right side of your brain behind.

How do you decide between trying to talk and listen to God by yourself or with others?

My goal is to be able to talk and listen to God anytime and anywhere by myself and with people, even if they are not trying to listen to God. However, sometimes I needed extra support dialoguing with God about painful situations. When it felt like I was stuck, I worked with a trustworthy listening coach who acted as my tow truck driver. I still stayed in the car with my hands on the wheel, but a coach took good notes and asked a few good questions while I interacted with God.

I believe it is crucial to be selective and cautious when working with a coach. With all the available methods, techniques, and training in praying for others, we can become over-reliant on others to do our work. Likewise, coaches who assert too much power or act with a sense of superiority can detract others from establishing their own connections with God. Unfortunately, I speak from more experience than I wish I had on both sides of this equation. However, this has driven me to learn how to go to God first and to do only what is needed to support others until they themselves can do the same.

Now if I feel a little stuck, it is more common for me to meet with a trusted person or small group and share a little about how I am feeling and why. When we take our time to listen to God individually and then share what we are sensing God saying, I become unstuck by listening both to what I am hearing and what my friend(s) are hearing. This is such a refreshing way of being a community of believers.

Where did you learn that? How do you know that? Where can I get that information?

I have thoroughly enjoyed translating the concepts I learned from neuroscience, psychology, and theology into terms and metaphors that fit with my ordinary life. I hope my book demonstrates how I have integrated what I learned and practiced from excellent resources. I chose not to distract from my heart-to-heart talks with God by citing research from those fields. If you are a little bit like me, you may feel tempted to flip to the resource list and start searching for a conference to attend, a speaker to listen to, or another book to buy. May I suggest that you first give yourself margin to reflect and interact with God about this book? Do you remember Tony's example from the introduction and chapter one?

Once you turn to the resource list, I especially recommend visiting the Immanuel Approach website since they guide you through the process of selecting resources that are best for you.[8]

How do I try this at home?

I hope you will draw your own conclusions and formulate your own plan for deepening your relationship with God as you are peeking in on my life with God. In the meantime, I will provide a brief overview of the habits that have most helped me these past four years.[9]

1. Get still and relax.

One of the most important things I have learned is how to relax my body for at least two minutes with exercises that are scientifically proven to calm our central nervous system.[10] Once my body is quiet, the chatter in my mind is also silenced, and my brain is unlocked with the discovery of a new thought. I believe God gives me new thoughts by showing me His perspective on me, life, and the world.

---

8. https://www.immanuelapproach.com/products-page/which-lehman-resources-are-right-for-me/

9. Steps two through five were developed by Dr. Karl Lehmann and are known as The Immanuel Approach. Lehmann, Karl, *The Immanuel Approach*, https://www.immanuelapproach.com/products-page/which-lehman-resources-are-right-for-me/
An asterisk in the resource list indicates resources that incorporate the Immanuel Approach in their training and materials. Please do remember to first discover what resources you and God have to access that are already in your heart! Take the time to respond to my book and get real with God first. After that, if you want to join me in an online small group to practice these steps go to https://deeperwalkinternational.org/journey for more information.

10. I love to coach clients in discovering their favorite relaxation exercises followed by practice in listening to God.

2. Ask God to help you think about a positive memory.[11]
I ask God to help me remember a time when I felt joy, peace, and the absence of pain, sadness, fear, or anxiety. It is great to start by thinking about a time when I was enjoying nature or something else beautiful and awe-inspiring. It could also be a time when I felt close to God.

3. Relive the memory for three minutes.
Once I land on a memory that fits this criteria, I set my timer for three minutes and relive it as if I were in an Imax theater. I journal, ask questions, describe details, and thank God out loud and in writing for the memory.

My conversations reveal the questions I asked, consistently proving and experiencing the discoveries in brain science—if we remain still and grateful for three minutes, our minds can conceive of a new thought and our spirits can see things from God's perspective. Now, for me, three minutes of silent appreciation feels like three seconds, and I am enticed to spend much more time interacting and learning from God about my own life and the impact of His faithful presence on my entire history. When I consider how God is present with every person that He ever created throughout all of time, it really helps me deal with despair about current events.

4. Interact with God about the memory.
Ask God lots of questions with the mindset that we don't want to overanalyze or use our sark. Instead, we want to see what God sees through His eyes and with our hearts. In the Bible, Paul refers to it as the *"eyes of your heart [the very center and core of your being]"* (Ephesians 1:18, Amplified). It has been so validating to realize that God sees every part of my history. God reminds me of things that were completely off my radar screen and then God

11. This is the hallmark of the Immanuel Approach.

shows me where He was and what He was doing. The fact that every part of my life is legitimate, has meaning, and provides an opportunity to learn and grow speaks volumes.

5. Write down everything you can about these interactions. I coach clients who have trouble staying focused to "*zoom in*" on that memory so it is all they see in their minds. Sometimes it helps to literally take our thumb and index finger and spread them apart as if we are enlarging something on a cell phone and to imagine we are enlarging the positive memory in our brain.

6. Practice, persevere, and be patient with the process. Commit to lifelong learning. I know what it is like to wonder, "Is this kind of intimacy with God reasonable to expect? Can this be real? I also remember sometimes feeling so tempted to revert to using prayer formulas or just going through the motions doing something that would look good to others. Being real with God, others, and ourselves is a very vulnerable place. I believe it is worth it.

Pause and ask yourself "how am I feeling after reading this book? I hope you are feeling courageous and convinced it is worth it. How desperate are you for a personal, interactive relationship with your Creator? Do you want this more than you want anything else in life? Are you convinced it is worth your focused attention and the opening up of your heart?

Are you sure that relaxation exercises are a Christian practice?

When I started learning how effective and scientifically valid relaxation exercises were, I was thrilled to see the integration of, and connection between, science and Christ-focused spirituality. I deeply appreciate how God designed our bodies, minds, and spirits to work together. The time is ripe for those of us whose bodies house the Holy Spirit to live like *"our bodies belong to the Lord"* rather than cutting ourselves off from them. *"The physical part of you is not some piece of property belonging to the spiritual part of you. God owns the whole works"* (1 Cor 6:19, MSG).

What if I try asking for a happy memory but can only remember negative ones?

Sometimes when I ask God to help me remember positive memories with feelings of peace and joy, negative parts of the memory emerge. I choose how to respond to that based on whether I felt overwhelmed or resilient. If I become too overwhelmed, I return to an established positive memory that gives me peace and joy, and I set aside the negative part for another time.

When I first started out, I spent months just focusing on positive memories. Once I felt enough strength, peace, and courage to stay curious when a mildly negative memory arose, I asked God questions such as, "How do you see this situation? What were you doing then? What do you want me to know? Why are you showing me this now? (The Glistening in chapter seven describes this type of experience.) This increased my resilience. This is a crucial point—as it became natural to converse with God in a present moment that felt negative, it felt safer and easier to chat with Him about a past moment that felt negative.

~~~

Where do I go from here?

I hope you will keep moving forward in the things that matter most in life no matter how difficult. I hope you will keep conversations with God, yourself, and others even when it is hard. Remember that your life is valuable and your mental and spiritual health is your greatest asset.
~~~

May I suggest forming some action steps around these categories:

1. Schedule time for real talk. Make an appointment in your calendar. If you already have the habit of a personal devotion, ask yourself: Do I schedule additional time for this or do I integrate this into what I am already doing?
2. Determine one concrete way of reminding yourself to talk with God anytime or anywhere. Is there a physical object you usually have with you that can gently nudge you to keep your heart open to God? Maybe it is something you put in your pocket, a piece of jewelry or a water bottle.
3. Keep a journal. Maybe you need an extra journal in your car or at work in a travel bag. I believe little notepads and post-it notes count as journals too. If you have given a really good try at responding with your heart and you want another resource, my top suggestion is *Joyful Journey*.
4. Find a healthy way of practicing real talk with God in a safe community. I would love to have you join me. To join an online small group that focuses on relational discipleship, listening to God, and listening to each other, you may request to work with me as your facilitator at: https://deeperwalkinternational.org/journey.
5. If you still feel the need for some outside support, please reach out to me for individualized coaching at lisadodgepinkham@gmail.com. Once I listen to your needs, desires, and goals, I will help you set up a great plan for realizing them. I aim to pay attention to you until you become an expert at paying attention to yourself and to provide enough support, structure, and accountability so that you are soon empowered to coach yourself.

Acknowledgments

I joyfully acknowledge:

My friends who are thoughtful, forgiving, adventurous, and who like to hang out with me and God. Many of you are from several other countries and all over the U.S. who participate with me in LK10 communities of practice and Deeper Walk International journey groups. I thank God for you and technology! I also love living in an era that embraces, trains, and values coaches, and I am thankful for all of you who have coached me these past four years. Readers, please check out their websites.

My two brilliant, creative, strong, and kind adult daughters who show me that God is *"compassionate and gracious, slow to anger, abounding in love and faithfulness"* (Psalm 86:15). It is an honor to be your mom, ladies!

My parents who always keep the porch light on. I hope my stories convey how deeply I appreciate and receive your love and devotion.

My husband who works hard, plays well and wants Jesus most of all. The day we met you said how much you valued your church community because they tried to be real. I feel grateful that we agree to *"let mutual love continue."* I feel hopeful as we learn how to be even more real with God, each other and the world.

My editor, Rachel McCracken, who created the right environment for me to risk sharing and improving my writing. Marcy Pusey—my enthusiastic and wise writing coach and Holly Duke—my dedicated, refreshing, and honest writing accountability partner.

My dear draft readers: Anita, Amy, Atara, Bill, David, Gillian, Jen, John, Laura, Lee, Mina, Steve, Tony and Wendi who generously gave their precious gifts of time, attention and honest feedback. Wow, my life is full of beautiful people. Thank you for your important and valuable contributions.

In a perfect world, we find the best mentors, internalize all that is good and pass it on. On this side of heaven, I must say that some of my most intimate encounters with Jesus, and my best learning and deepest transformations emerge from experiences I would never want to repeat. For all those who have involved me in those situations, I am grateful for what you taught me and how it drove me to God for His perspective, comfort, and validation.

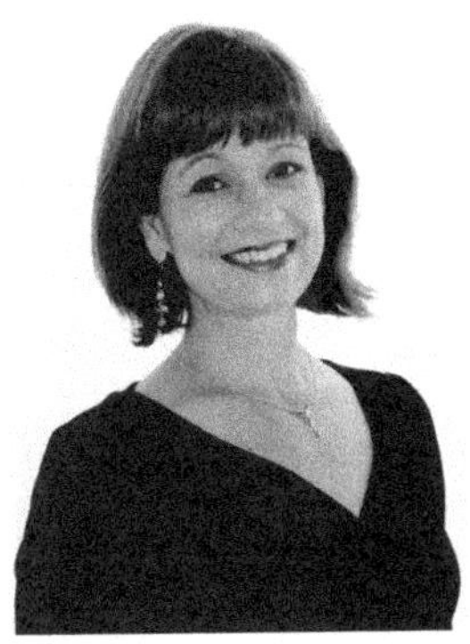

About the Author

Lisa Dodge Pinkham is passionate about fostering intimate and authentic relationships with God. She is a leadership coach and certified health coach who has helped individuals, couples, families, and small groups achieve their optimum level of health in all aspects of life for over thirty years.

She works with people all over the world who are seeking to develop healthy Christian communities. Her previous vocations include campus ministry, speaking, teaching, homeschooling, curriculum writing, and leadership development.

Pinkham graduated from Gordon-Conwell Seminary with a Master of Art in Religion with a concentration in Adult Education. She graduated University of New Hampshire majoring in Exercise Physiology with minors in Psychology and Dance.

She recently completed basic through advanced training in the Immanuel Approach with Dr. Karl Lehmann and is currently training/being trained with Deeper Walk International, Life Model Works and the LK10 Community. Pinkham aspires to integrate Christian spiritual disciplines, neuroscience, and total health making that easily accessible to everyone.

A native New Englander, she currently resides in Kent Island, Maryland, with her husband of twenty-six years. She has two amazing, grown daughters and enjoys singing, dancing, spending time in nature, and traveling—even on road trips.

Resources

Contact me:

To join an online small group that focuses on relational discipleship, listening to God and listening to each other, you may request to work with me as your facilitator at https://deeperwalkinternational.org/journey. For individualized coaching, contact me at lisa@lisadodgepinkham.com. Once I listen to your needs, desires, and goals, I will help you set up a great plan for realizing them.

Books:

- Brown, Amy, and Chris Coursey. *Brain Skills in the Bible: A Transforming Fellowship Bible Study*. CreateSpace Independent Publishing Platform, 2018.
- Brown, Brene. *Braving the Wilderness: The Quest for True Belonging and the Courage to Stand Alone*. N.Y., N.Y.: Penguin Random House, 2017.

- Coursey, Chris. *Transforming Fellowship: 19 Brain Skills That Build Joyful Community*. East Peoria, Ill.: Shepherd's House, 2016.
- Daniels, David, and Virginia Price. *The Essential Enneagram.* N.Y., N.Y.: Harper Collins, 2009.
- Daniels, Toni. *Back to Joy: An Intimate Journey with Jesus into Emotional Health and Maturity.* Self-Publishing School, 2016.
- Friesen, James, James Wilder, Anne Bierling, Rick Koepcke, and Maribeth Poole. *Living from the Heart Jesus Gave You.* East Peoria, Ill: Shepherd's House, 2013.
- Lehmann, Karl, *The Immanuel Approach.*
  Please visit the website as it is designed to help the reader choose the resources that would be most helpful. https://www.immanuelapproach.com/products-page/which-lehman-resources-are-right-for-me/
  I especially appreciate this diagram that depicts the Immanuel Approach towards conversations with God. https://lifemodelworks.azureedge.net/wp-content/uploads/2018/08/Immanuel-Healing-God-With-Us.pdf
- Linn, Matthew, Sheila Fabricant Linn, and Dennis Linn. *Healing Spiritual Abuse and Religious Addiction.* Mahwah, N.J.: Paulist Press, 1994.
- Parry, Alan, and Linda Parry. *Where Is Jesus?* Carol Stream, Ill.: Tyndale Kids, 1998.
- Rath, Tom. *Strengthsfinder 2.0.* N.Y., N.Y.: Gallup Press, 2007.
- Rohr, Richard. *Falling Upward: A Spirituality for the Two Halves of Life*. San Fra, Ca.: Jossey -Bass, 2011.
- Rohr, Richard. *The Art of Letting Go*. Sounds True, 2010, Audiobook.
- Smith, Kent. *Centered*, JFN Resources, 2009.

- Stalcup, Betsy. Immanuel DVD, https://www.godhealstoday.org/products#anchor-link-Immanuel-DVD
- Thompson, Curt, MD. *Anatomy of the Soul*. Carrollton, TX: Tyndale, 2010.
- Wilder, James, Ed Khouri, Chris Coursey, and Sheila Sutton. *Joy Starts Here: The Transformation Zone*. East Peoria, Ill: Shepherd's House, 2013.
  To download Chapter ten of *Joy Starts Here* for free click here: http://www.joy2thrive.com/PDF/JSH_chapter10.pdf
- Wilder, James, Anna Kang, John Loppnow, and Sungshim Loppnow. *Joyful Journey*. East Peoria, Ill.: Shepherd's House, 2015. I especially appreciate this journaling template from Joyful Journey. https://lifemodelworks.azureedge.net/wp-content/uploads/2018/08/Joyful-Journey-Questions.pdf

Websites

- Life Model Works: To explore the books and workbooks that I used personally and in classes, see the list of top seller books here: https://shop.lifemodelworks.org/collections/top-sellers-books.
  This includes Connexus Classes (weekly for twelve weeks): Belonging, Forming, Restarting and Life Model Works Thrive Training (Week long intensives)
- Daniels, Matt, and Toni Daniels. Transforming Conflict. https://www.transformingconflict.io/.
- Deeper Walk International: Journey Groups. https://deeperwalkinternational.org/journey/

You may request to participate in a group with me as your group leader. Journey groups provide learning content and a small group to practice the concepts developed by Life Model Works, the Immanuel Approach and LK10.

- Jones, Darrin, and Julie Jones. Golden Goose Consulting. https://www.goldengooseconsulting.com/.
- LK10 Community: Church 101 & Leader Teams. https://lk10.com/.
- Loppnow, John, and Sungshim Loppnow. *"Presence and Practice."* Presence and Practice. https://www.presenceand-practice.com/. Co-Authors of Joyful Journey.
- Morris, Tim, and Brittani Morris. Design Discovery. https://designdiscovery.com/. Design Discovery Coaching
- Stosny, Steven, PhD. Compassion Power. http://www.compassionpower.com/.
- Yerkovich, Mylan, and Kay Yerkovich. How We Love. https://howwelove.com/.

TED Talks

- Achor, Shawn. *"The Happy Secret to Better Work."* TedTalk. 2011. https://www.ted.com/talks/shawn_achor_the_happy_secret_to_better_work.
- Brown, Brene. *"Listening to Shame."* TedTalk. 2012. https://www.ted.com/talks/brene_brown_listening_to_shame/transcript?language=en.
- Brown, Brene. *"The Power of Vulnerability."* TedTalk. 2010. https://www.ted.com/talks/brene_brown_on_vulnerability?language=en.

YouTube:

Please enjoy this great variety of songs with both a sense of humor and worship!

- Blue, Suede. *"Hooked on a Feeling."* YouTube. https://www.youtube.com/watch?v=Bo-qweh7nbQ.
- Baloche, Paul. *"Open the Eyes of My Heart."* YouTube. https://www.youtube.com/watch?v=ViBNqNukgzE
- Card, Michael. *"Arise My Love."* YouTube. https://www.youtube.com/watch?v=o29wibpA4RQ.
- Croce, Jim. *"I Have to Say I Love You in a Song."* YouTube. https://www.youtube.com/watch?v=EN1nMpmC0n4.
- Eldridge, John. *"Walking With God."* YouTube. https://www.youtube.com/watch?v=TWgl7oOzM04.
- Franklin, Aretha. *"Freeway of Love."* YouTube. https://www.youtube.com/watch?v=Ip_pjb5_fgA.
- Haydn, Franz J. *"Sing a New Song to the Lord."* YouTube. https://www.youtube.com/watch?v=sWq2PbrIXWw.
- Take 6. *"I LOVE You."* YouTube. https://www.youtube.com/watch?v=smRcxpBdk04.
- Miles, Charles Austin. *"I Come to the Garden Alone."* YouTube. https://www.youtube.com/watch?v=NQ2Mcd7pX20.
- Nash, Johnny. *"I Can See Clearly Now."* YouTube. https://www.youtube.com/watch?v=FscIgtDJFXg.
- Taylor, James. *"Something in the Way She Moves."* YouTube. https://www.youtube.com/watch?v=Bfk9nvUni88. (My husband imagines this song is about Holy Spirit.)
- The Temptations. *"Ain't Too Proud to Beg."* YouTube. https://www.youtube.com/watch?v=3s0TkufXA38.
- Timberlake, Justin. *"Can't Stop the Feeling."* YouTube. https://www.youtube.com/watch?v=ru0K8uYEZWw. Consider this your invitation to dance wherever you are!
- Tomlin, Chris. *"Enough."* YouTube. https://www.youtube.com/watch?v=87Ig-lnWjzQ.

Movies

- Frozen. By Hans Christian Andersen. Screenplay by Jennifer Lee. Performed by Jennifer Lee, Chris Buck. IMDB. https://www.imdb.com/title/tt2294629/?ref_=fn_al_tt_1.
- Inside Out. Screenplay by Pete Docter. Directed by Ronnie Del Carmen. Performed by Amy Poehler, Phyllis Smith. IMDB. https://www.imdb.com/title/tt2096673/.
  This is a very creative, humorous and evocative demonstration of the application of brain science in family life.
- Groundhog Day. Screenplay by Danny Rubin and Harold Ramis. Performed by Bill Murray, Andie MacDowell. IMDB. https://www.imdb.com/title/tt0107048/.

Contact Me:

In case you missed this earlier, here it is again.

To join an online small group that focuses on relational discipleship, listening to God and listening to each other, you may request to work with me as your facilitator at https://deeperwalk-international.org/journey. For individualized coaching contact me at lisa@lisadodgepinkham.com. Once I listen to your needs, desires, and goals, I will help you set up a great plan for realizing them.